𝒏ot
THE
MILKY WAY

By Dr. Ravpreet Singh

Copyright © 2023 by Dr. Ravpreet Singh
All rights reserved.
This book or any portion thereof may not be reproduced or used in any manner whatsoever without the express written permission of the respective writer of the respective content except for the use of brief quotations in a book review.
The writer of the respective work holds sole responsibility for the originality of the content and The Write Order is not responsible in any way whatsoever.
Printed in India
ISBN: 978-93-5776-333-2
First Printing, 2023

The Write Order Publications
Koramangala, Bangalore
Karnataka-560029
www.thewriteorder.com

Typeset by Shreshta Veergandham
Publishing Consultant- Aishwarya
Book Cover designed by Manaswani K Saxena

DISCLAIMER

The information presented in this book is completely based on personal observations and clinical experience. Hurting anyone's personal or financial matters is not what is intended. The intention here is to advise readers about a good and healthy lifestyle and prevent getting a few major diseases even after having a strong family history of the same disease. It is important for the readers to understand that all humans are different and have different body types and tendencies, and there is no 'one rule that applies to all'. Some readers might feel the information to be a little overwhelming and contrary to what has been believed for many years, so the only way out is to try following what is said as an experiment. For at least two to three months and see the results for yourself. If you still feel you do not feel better, you can always and again switch back to the previous routine. It is probably then you will realize the actual difference. The good or bad effects might not be evident immediately, but I am certain that most of you will benefit from this book. Or at least I hope so.

IT'S NOT THE TRUTH THAT WE SEEK
IT'S WHAT IS BELIEVABLE

CONTENTS

1. INTRODUCTION 1

2. HISTORY 7

3. DO WE NEED MILK AS OUR DAILY DRINK ? 13

4. WITHOUT RENNIN, YOU ARE JUST A FART MACHINE! ... 20

5. THE MINDSET- IT'S PRIDE AND NOT PROTEIN 25

6. STOP BLAMING YOUR GENES 27

7. FIGHT OR FLIGHT RESPONSE IN MR. RAHUL's CASE 35

8. THE STRANGE CASE OF HYPOCALCEMIA 39

9. MALE BREASTS AND FEMALE BEARD 44

10. WHY LACTOSE INTOLERANCE IS A "BLESSING IN DISGUISE" 47

11. PROBLEM WITH MILK PROTEINS 52

12. OXYTOCIN- A LIFE SAVING DRUG, STILL GOT BANNED. WHY? 58

13. WHAT IS BST? WHAT IS RECOMBINANT BST? 61

14. CAN HUMANS REALLY DIGEST MILK COMPLETELY? 66

15. WHAT IS COMMON IN THYROID, PCOD AND DIABETES? 71

16. CAN STOPPING DAIRY ACTUALLY REVERSE MAJOR DISEASES? 74

17. INSULIN AND DAIRY 78

18. GLOBAL WARMING DUE TO MILK? 82

19. WHAT IS THE ALTERNATIVE 90

20. IS ANIMAL CRUELTY THE ONLY REASON? 93

21. PITUITARY SHIT- UITARY GLAND 96

22. END NOTE 99

"AUDE SAPERE"

DARE TO BE WISE

Introduction

In the 2nd century AD, one of the most influential astronomer and geographer of that time proposed a theory. A theory that adhered to the religious beliefs that strongly believed about the Earth's centrality in the universe. The astronomer was well-known at the time, and his theory was extremely compelling. The name of the theory was 'Geocentric theory', and his name was Ptolemy of Alexandria.

The theory stated that "Earth is at the center of the universe and all the other planets, sun and stars revolve around the Earth."

His theory, in fact, was so compelling that the greatest of minds of that time, like Aristotle, was convinced to believe in that theory.

The world believed in that theory for whopping 1400 years. Just imagine how many generations have passed believing in this theory. This theory was taught in schools and colleges for years; the world believed in something that was not correct for hundreds of years. These were proposed by the men of science, smart people.

The world so strongly adopted the theory, by the scientists and churches both, that if anyone said anything against it, were punished.

In the year 1616, Galileo Galilei, who was also one

of the greatest minds ever in the history of mankind, was hanged to death on the charge of Heresy, which means a person who opposed the teachings of the church. The Church, at that time, believed in the Theory of Geocentrism. He was literally hanged because he said Earth revolved around the sun and not the other way around (which was the prevalent theory at that time). He was also not completely right, but what he said was much more logical than what the world believed.

The theory of Geocentrism was basically incorrect. So when the maximum population believed in that theory, then anyone who did not have knowledge about the same started believing in it too. After many years, a few curious minds who had the questioning mind started working on this concept and completely overturned it.

In the 15th century, a mathematician and astronomer, Nicolaus Copernicus was the one who gave the theory of "Heliocentrism."

He was the mind behind Galileo's statement, who got hanged because of being correct scientifically.

The theory of Heliocentrism states- that "It's, not the earth that is the center of the universe, but it's the Sun." This was a major upgrade to the last geocentric theory. But still, this theory was also not completely correct. But it changed a lot of things in the scientific world. And yes, science is an evolving subject; we have been able to discover and invent wonders.

And, then, after a few hundred years, came an another theory that said it is neither the sun nor the earth that is the center of the universe. In fact, astronomers discovered something completely different, which was supported by mathematical calculations, The Big Bang

Theory, which said that the universe started as a single huge explosion and is still expanding to date. This theory is still believed to be the most appropriate theory at present, or we can say it's our best guess at present.

Why this fact needs a mention here because there might be a possibility of whatever you thought was right (scientifically) for your entire life can still be wrong, factually. Just because our parents or grandparents or great grand parents consumed milk and cottage cheese through their entire life and thought that it was really good for health or had a lot of calcium, doesn't mean they were right. They never got the ingredients checked. And if they relied only on their observation, sadly, they were pretty bad at it. Why they started having it in the first place is a different matter altogether that goes back thousands of years, which I will discuss later in the history chapter.

They thought they got immunity from cow's milk, in fact, they might have got it from their own mother's milk at a very younger age because most of us get our immunity from that source, called acquired immunity, and another immunity is innate immunity, which is our immunity by birth. They were probably wrong there.

They also might have thought milk made them stronger, but in fact, the strength they had might have been from the natural and less preserved vegetables they had at that time, which we don't get easily nowadays. And a much more physically active lifestyle, which, we don't get any more in our sedentary and indoor, air-conditioned jobs. So they might have misjudged it in this case also. Because I got convinced by one thing that I will explain here in this book, and I am hopeful that this will be helpful to all the readers too.

Okay, so MILK.

We all know what it is, the first thing that enters our body when we enter the world when we are born. Our very first food, food that helps us grow as an infant, helps us attain immunity, and gives us antibiotic-like antibodies, which gives us strength to fight all the infections as an infant when we are fragile, weak, and vulnerable. The first milk that mammals produce after giving birth to their younger ones is called Colostrum. It is most rich in antibodies and has a much higher concentration of fats and proteins as compared to milk coming after 4-8 days of birth. That's why the term 'First Milk' has huge importance in the dairy world.

Newborns have very immature and small digestive systems, and colostrum delivers its nutrients in a very concentrated, low-volume form. It has a mild laxative effect, encouraging the passing of the baby's first stool, which is called meconium. This clears excess bilirubin, a waste product of dead red blood cells produced in large quantities at birth due to blood volume reduction from the infant's body and helps prevent jaundice. Colostrum is known to contain immune cells (as lymphocytes) and many antibodies such as IgA, IgG, and IgM. These are some of the components of the adaptive immune system.

Mothers milk- First milk (colostrum) or the milk coming after that is the most important food for the infant.

Quick question, Why is human milk good and cow's milk bad?

Answer- Cow's milk is also good, but only for their babies. Human milk is good for human babies.

The fact that milk is good for human beings has a big question mark. At least I see it, but many of you might not see it. The point is, are we ready to accept it? Accept the fact that the entire human civilisation did not observe its bad effects for so many years. Drinking milk might have had a completely different approach towards the animals and milk requirements back then when humans started drinking milk.

So, a few curious questions,

When did we (humans) first start drinking milk?

Why did we start having milk at all?

What lead us to do that?

Answer- This happened in the Neolithic Era (Era of Agriculture Revolution), An era which is identified as when life was nomadic, when we were wanderers, hopping from one place to another hoping for better food and shelter. An era when we first thought settling was a better option than wandering. And then we had to grow food where we lived, so we learned how to do that. Plus, anything that tasted normal and didn't kill us was food back then- meat, beef, milk, chicken, fish, plants etc.

Humans started experimenting with crop growing in this era, which is also called an era of the agricultural revolution. We started drinking milk out of necessity because of the very limited food options that we had at that time. Back then, nobody cared how much calcium or protein it had or how many calories it might give us. There were no ways to calculate such parameters. It was not a business then, but sadly, it is now, so we need to project it as the healthiest drink, and advertise it as the only source of calcium because we need to sell it.

Always remember we did not start drinking milk because it was healthy, we started drinking milk, and then we started projecting it as a healthy drink. We definitely need to know more about the history of why and when exactly humans started having milk or extracting milk from other animals.

History

Humans started consuming dairy products during the NEOLITHIC REVOLUTION, also known as the AGRICULTURAL REVOLUTION, which was wide -a scale transition of many human cultures from a lifestyle of hunting and gathering to one of agriculture and settlement, making an increasingly larger population possible. It is imperative that we know the history of why at all we started having milk.

We first domesticated the most important dairy animals- cattle, sheep and goats- in Southwest Asia. However, domestic cattle had been independently derived from wild Aurochs (a large, black European wild Ox. Extinct since 1627) populations several times since.

Initially, animals were kept for meat, and archaeologist Andrew Sherratt has suggested that dairying, along with the exploitation of domestic animals for hair and labor, began much later in a separate secondary products revolution in the fourth millennium BC.

But Sherratt's model is not supported by recent findings, based on the analysis of lipid residue in prehistoric pottery, that show that dairying was practised in the early phases of agriculture in Southwest Asia by at least the seventh millennium BC.

Camels, domesticated in central Arabia in the fourth millennium BC, have also been used as dairy animals in North Africa and the Arabian Peninsula. The earliest Egyptian records of burn treatments describe burn dressings using milk from mothers of male babies. In the rest of the world (i.e., East and Southeast Asia, the Americas and Australia), milk and dairy products were historically not a large part of the diet, either because they remained populated by hunter-gatherers who did not keep animals or the local agricultural economies did not include domesticated dairy species. Milk consumption became common in these regions comparatively recently as a consequence of European colonialism and political domination over much of the world in the last 500 years.

It was only after the settled communities and colonies were formed we started learning new things.

This was the first time in human history that these settled communities learned to experiment with plants and crop growing.

This was the time when humans started domestication of animals too. The archaeological data suggests that this kind of domestication of plants and animals took place in various parts of the world around 12000 years ago, independently. It was a 'first of its kind" revolution.

It was a revolution, no doubt about it, but it came with its downside too. Many good things happened to humanity after that, or at least we like to think it that way. In a way, humans learned to 'live in a community, like a community', for good. This gave them an immense sense of security at various levels. They marked their territories, made houses and colonies. Learned to adjust to the weather changes and safety from wild animals also there was a big jump in the security of their family, especially children. Earlier, kids used to be a burden, because carrying a small child with you while hunting and gathering must have been a problematic task. Secure houses and living in one place solved that problem.

But, it gave rise to a different set of new problems that humanity is still suffering from and paying its cost. The previous lifestyle was a much more active, physically tiring lifestyle. They were always on the move, climbing trees, and eating fresh fruits and wild figs, which kept them strong and healthy.

Compared to the settled lifestyle, their tasks changed from climbing trees to taking care of the crops they were growing, watering them, sowing and plucking. Most of these tasks required bending of their backs. A study of the ancient skeletons showed that this revolution gave humans diseases like arthritis, disc degeneration, and hernias. If milk had all the calcium they needed, joint pains should have been the last disease they suffered from. Because that's what we believe these days. Have pain in your joints, start taking calcium supplements.

It doesn't end here. After growing crops, they stored them, without having the right knowledge and resources for it. It took them time to learn it, but they got sick frequently because of this reason too. Also, stored and cooked food was less nutritious as compared to the fresh fruits and figs that they consumed in the hunting lifestyle.

All the back pains and different joint troubles are very individual problems, as not everyone suffers from them. It depends on the body type, strength, genetics and resistance also. And at that time, the good part about it was these were not contagious problems. Some suffered from it, and many managed to avoid it.

But when we mention contagious diseases, agricultural revolution was the Dark Age of disease and human suffering. When these settled communities domesticated animals, they had to take care of them. Washing them, milking them, cleaning their excreta etc., exposed them to a galore of new infections.

There was a cattle disease called Rinderpest, which started at that time only which used to be an endemic disease.

It was also known as the "Cattle Plague". It was a severely fatal disease, and in some herds, the death rate was hundred per cent.

It infected only the cattle and is believed to have jumped from cattle to humans in the form of Measles. Just like Covid-19 is believed to be transferred to humans from bats. Rinderpest was believed to be a cousin of Measles. And we all are well aware of the fact that, even a thousand years later today, measles is still around, and even after decades of vaccination, we are unable to eradicate it.

Many scientists believed that diseases like measles, mumps, scarlet fever, diphtheria, and whooping cough only started during the time of this revolution. And similarly, these diseases are still around.

Also, when any herd or community got infected by any of these contagious diseases, they thought it was a curse from some God. And with no medication or no knowledge of how to deal with that situation, the only solution they had at that time was to leave the place and shift to a new place or join another community in the vicinity. Which, conclusively only helped the infection to spread to various new places. And this led to the spread of these infections around the world.

As time passed, the number of diseases and cases increased. What initially looked like a BOON to humanity, the safety of kids and security turned into BANE when the infant mortality rate started increasing. When obesity, diabetes and cardiovascular disease hit the communities. Several ethnological and archaeological studies also suggest that cereal-based diet and sedentary lifestyle also added to the reduction in life expectancy and stature.

Why Neolithic revolution deserves mention in this book is because it was this time when humans started domesticating animals, and that led to the suffering from communicable diseases, specifically those they got from animals, such as influenza, measles, smallpox etc., possible reasons at that time could be inadequate sanitary habits, eating meat and having milk of the animals with very limited knowledge of the diseases these mammals could have been suffering from, at that time.

We already had a list of causes that we knew caused these diseases, and I am just adding something to that list. And that might not change a lot in history but it may bring a big change in our lives in the coming future.

Starting to consume dairy products was right or wrong?

Agricultural revolution was good or bad, depends on what's your opinion about it. But one thing is for sure. It gave rise to many problems that we still are figuring out solutions to.

Conclusion- Humans did not start having milk in search of calcium but this is what is implied these days everywhere. In fact, they did it because of lack of eating options when they started to settle in one place and changed their lifestyle from being hunter-gatherers to settled communities.

Do We Need Milk As Our Daily Drink?

Humans are the only species of mammals who derive and drink milk from other mammals for the requirement or, according to me, the obsession of getting more calcium, right? Or getting stronger bones, maybe, right? These questions led me to search for the animals or mammals having the strongest bones. It turns out that "the femur of the Rhino" is considered to be the strongest bone in the world. Also, heavy animals like elephants and horses have strong weight-bearing bones. And I haven't seen any of these animals drinking cow's milk or milk from any other animal to get stronger bones. Ironically, all these stronger animals are completely Herbivores, which means (of course, you know what it means) that they eat only plants or fruits. In human nomenclature, they are Vegetarians or Vegans.

The amount of calcium that is there in our bones or blood directly depends on two things, vitamin-D levels and parathyroid hormone.

Parathyroid hormone is the only hormone solely responsible for the regulation of calcium levels in our blood and bones. It is secreted by parathyroid glands, which are 4 in number, and present behind the thyroid gland. Our obsession with calcium intake or milk drinking might not make any sense if we do not have sufficient parathormone in our bodies. Even though it is rare that this hormone decreases. High levels of parathormone are more common. But if you have normal levels of this hormone, and have a normal diet that includes vegetables or fruits in it, then you might not have to worry about your calcium levels.

Myth Buster- Milk is considered the most healthy drink, it has a lot of calcium, proteins and a lot of other nutrients in it. It makes you stronger and healthier etc. We were grown up seeing advertisements saying how healthy milk is. That happy face of the child standing with a smiling cow gives us an impression of how happy the cow is at the dairy farms, which I believe is far away from the reality. All of us know about the reality of their conditions. Many undercover videos have been released to show how they are treated there. Obviously, it is inhuman to do any kind of harm to any animal or human. But, it's not only about that, but it is also about, is it really good for you? Do you think human civilisation could NOT have survived without it? Can we not derive all the ingredients present in milk from any other source? Does milk have anything really exclusive in it? The answer to all these questions is probably NO.

These Advertisements were imprinted in my mind so deeply that even after observing and knowing how harmful it is for us, I was not convinced completely that even I used to ask this question to myself that, "Wait, am I sure about this?", "Is it actually healthy to quit having milk or dairy products?" what about my body's calcium requirement? I don't want to take calcium pills for my entire life. How will I be able to match my calcium requirement? These are all the obvious questions popping up in everyone's mind as soon as I ask anyone to stop dairy. Fear of getting diseased is the fear we all have had or have at some point of time in our lives. No one wants to be unhealthy or sick. But we don't need to fear it; we just need to have the knowledge of how to prevent it. Nobody likes to go to a doctor; everyone goes when they need to. Consider this a life hack to prevent going to a doctor, but unfortunately, our thinking is the other way around.

But, What about the people who choose not to drink milk?

Either they don't like it, or they cannot simply digest it. Are they not healthy? Or do they die early? Do they die of hypocalcaemia (a condition of calcium deficiency)? Can anyone actually die of hypocalcaemia? answer to all these questions is also NO. You all know that. You don't need to hear this from anyone else.

Can they not survive without it? Also, are they more prone to fractures or joint troubles? But as a fact, people who have regular milk can also suffer from calcium deficiency. Did you know, excessive consumption of coffee and alcohol also leads to calcium deficiency? And it is even more harmful than coffee and alcohol, But how many of us will actually stop drinking coffee or alcohol after reading this? Hardly anyone. So it's time we should stop killing other animals just for a little bit of calcium, which we might get from plenty of other sources, without killing anyone.

In fact, milk is not the only source of calcium we have. We have much better options, that have much more calcium than milk. And options that will not give you diseases like Thyroid or PCOD, heart conditions etc. That will not give you gastritis, or bloating. Or will not make you fat. Or will not give you unnecessary hormone imbalances.

Being in medical practice gives us exposure to knowing about the lives and experiences of many people. To observe and learn many things in our practice, that we never learn during our academic times in our college, It is a lot different when you sit at your clinic. One important thing that I have observed in my practice is that the first thing that comes to people's minds when they experience joint pain or body pain is, a deficiency of calcium, which is not entirely true. In fact, a commonest cause of joint pain diagnostically is OA or RA. That is, osteoarthritis or rheumatoid arthritis, and in both these problems you will find a family tendency or hereditary tendency to get the disease. OA generally affects old age people, commonly after the age of 40 years, due to overuse or wear and tear of the joints. RA can happen at any age and is more common in women than men. Both these diseases have actually very less to do with our calcium consumption. But let us not get too carried away, calcium is really important for our body, That is also an undeniable fact. But, we all really need to get over the thought process that, it is the only cause of joint pains. And if anyone of you really had calcium for treating joint pains, ask yourself, did having calcium tablets really cure you from the joint pains? I doubt it.

Medically, all of us should consult an Orthopedician before starting calcium or any other supplement for pains in joints or the body, and not self-diagnose ourselves. Or, at least get the calcium tested through a simple blood test and then start the supplement, that too after consulting a professional.

By definition, milk is a nutrient-rich, white liquid food produced by the mammary glands of mammals, to feed their infant mammals before they are able to digest other food. Early lactation milk by mother mammals contains colostrum, which contains the mother's antibodies, and helps the infant mammal to gain better immunity. It's a known fact in human infants that, kids who take mother's milk have better immunity than infants who are not able to take mother's milk.

But it's a lesser-known fact that mammals can not completely digest milk extracted, from other mammals. Naturally, it is meant for their own infant mammals.

Has anyone tried giving a glass of human milk to a calf? Doesn't that sound funny to you? I am sure it is equally weird for the cows also when they go through all the forceful milk extraction process at the dairy farm. Just kidding...!!! Cows don't have a sense of humor, only humans are blessed with it, but that doesn't mean they don't have feelings. Many pieces of research have proved that cows staying in farms who are forced to lactate suffer from stress and depression.

Data says dairy farms produced 730 million tones of milk in the year 2011, from 260 million dairy cows, that's a lot of depressed cows. India is the largest producer of milk and a leading exporter of skimmed milk powder. And, throughout the world, more than six billion people are estimated to consume milk and milk products.

For thousands of years milk is considered to be the best food, it is considered a holy drink in some places. The cow is a holy animal, in my country, so cows milk has to be holy and helpful to humans, even cows urine is believed to cure some diseases, but many scientists don't support the idea of the medicinal abilities of cow's urine as there is no sturdy scientific research supporting this hypothesis. But Even to this day, many still believe this.

Also, What I fail to understand is that, how can you abuse someone for milk, and call them your God at the same time?

There is a growing observation of people becoming intolerant to milk or lactose or any kind of dairy product. They are just unable to digest either all or any particular milk product. Did this happen suddenly? If yes, then how is it possible, that someone who was used to drinking milk since childhood, and suddenly stopped digesting it or started having trouble digesting it? So what went wrong? Where or when did it go wrong?

Many theories are being postulated these days on what is wrong with milk. Why are dairy products so harmful? Are they only harmful to cows or buffaloes, or also to humans...? why are they harming us now, or were they always harmful? Can humans really digest cow's or buffalo's milk?

There are many questions like these, which came to my mind when I started looking for answers and started advising my patients to at least try stopping dairy products for the given conditions, and with no surprise, almost everyone got benefitted from it. I, not being the first one to enlighten about the bad effects of dairy or animal products, admit that, the more I gained knowledge about dairy products, the more I hated them because it is harmful to both, us and the cattle. And also for the environment.

I am fortunate enough that I got the opportunity to treat a large number of patients having gastric troubles. I always guide them with dietary changes, lifestyle changes, and sticking to the routine to avoid hyperacidity or reflux or heartburn or gastritis, along with the medicines. But cutting their dairy products has helped them a lot, in relieving gastritis or bloating. If you haven't tried this, you should.

Basically, lactose in milk products is digested by an enzyme called lactase in humans and we need rennin and pepsin in our body to digest milk proteins. Will explain these in detail, later. But it is important first to know what lactose intolerance is. (details later)

Without Rennin, You Are Just A Fart Machine!

Rennin or Chymosin is a proteolytic enzyme related to pepsin that is synthesized by chief cells in the stomach of some animals. Its role in digestion is to curdle or coagulate milk in the stomach, a process of considerable importance in very young animal.

In a nutshell, A- it is the mandatory enzyme, which is required to digest milk proteins, specifically casein protein. It converts liquid milk into solid milk, curd or cheese-like material in our stomach. B- also helps in the production of cheese.

But obviously, there's more to it, and the story is not a happy one.

When I first thought of digestive enzymes or rennin, I thought, textbooks of our medical college or biology school books must have had some sort of mention in them. As the only "renin" word I remembered was in the Renin-Angiotensin mechanism. Which is not the same as Rennin or Rennet.

"Rennin", or "Chymosin" or "Rennet" I couldn't recall. So I had to look it up in the books. The only thing mentioned was, "Humans do not have Rennin in their body, and it is a milk-curdling enzyme". This basically means that we cannot either completely or partially digest Casein protein, which forms the major part of the milk protein content because without rennin we cannot break casein protein. And yes we do have an enzyme to help digest casein protein, but not as quickly as done by rennin, it takes hours to break casein, the reason for the slow digestion of milk.

In order to understand how Chymosin coagulates the milk, one needs to know something about milk proteins. The majority of milk proteins is Casein and it is a slow-digesting protein. Other details about this protein will be in later in the chapter, problems with milk proteins.

Human milk has approximately 60% casein protein and 40% whey protein, while cow's milk has 80% casein and 20% whey protein. And the problem with casein is that all of us cannot digest it. In fact, most of us cannot digest it at all, and some of us can digest it a little. But even though 60% of casein is present in human milk, how is that digested?

First of all, we all have human's or mother's milk during the first 2-3 years of our life. Because human infants do have a pseudo rennin or chymosin-like an enzyme that helps them digest casein present in their mother's milk. This enzyme starts depleting after we wean off.

Surprisingly, this topic is under-researched, in the context of the enormous usage of milk and dairy products and also in the context of the number of questions asked considering the benefits of dairy products. It is not well researched by coincidence or deliberately, I don't know.

Very few articles had information on whether humans have rennin or not, but every article knew for sure that a cow's fourth abdomen had plenty of good quality rennet in it, which helps in curdling the milk and production of cheese.

Casein protein is a very commonly used protein in the bodybuilding world. Some gym instructors advise casein protein as a supplement while bodybuilding as it remains in our stomach for a longer time because it is a comparatively slow-digesting protein. And according to them, it promotes muscle growth.

But, anything that stays longer in your stomach will ultimately generate more stress on your digestive enzymes, coming from the pancreas or gall bladder, leading to unnecessary stress on the pancreas leading it to malfunction. Conclusively, over utilizing the insulin of your body increasing your blood glucose levels and may increase your chances of suffering from diseases like Diabetes.

While humans can digest whey protein in cow's milk, we cannot completely digest casein, and this is where the issue lies. Without the help of Rennin, to digest casein, it becomes indigestible and even poisonous. Reference(www.anoasisofhealing.com).

It is pepsin which helps our body to digest proteins, and all proteins are not alike, we have thousands of types of proteins in our body, which helps us in various kind of functions, and in fact, in almost every kind of activity, proteins are required.

Humans can digest humans milk easily, because, naturally, our digestive system is made to do that, as we have only one stomach. Do you knowhow many stomachs a cow has?

Four.

Yes, it is called a Ruminant stomach- mammals like cows, goats, sheep, camel, pigs, etc are cud-chewing mammals. All animals of these kinds have four stomachs: RUMEN, RETICULUM, OMASUM AND ABOMASUM. Out of all these, the fourth one i.e Abomasum, is the most important in digesting milk. Because it contains Renin in it. And without renin it's impossible to digest cow's milk.

And all the cud-chewing animals have a completely different process of digestion than humans because the food they swallow after eating once comes back to their mouth for chewing again and swallowing the second time.

In 1935, two doctors did a study on the amount of time humans take to digest various food items.

Dr Maile and Dr Scott did the experiment on three doctors, their wives, one dentist and one medical student. Surprisingly, milk was found to be one of the most tedious food items to be digested. It took them six and a half hours to digest only a pint of milk. Whereas, only 3-4 hours to digest an ordinary meal.

So, almost a hundred years ago, it was scientifically proven that for humans, milk will not be easy to digest. And yet some people think, we have been drinking it for thousand years, and nothing wrong happened to us.

So, understanding the chronology here is important. Because what would you as a company do, if you came to know about something like this, obviously you will start adding substances to it to make it easily digestible, and if I say, it doesn't have enough calcium, then you will start fortifying milk with calcium too, and again if I say it doesn't have vitamin D in it, then, of course, you will fortify it with vitamin D. There is nothing wrong in adding minerals and vitamins in a product to sell it. The problem is in saying it is the only source of calcium and also not admitting to the fact that it is done by hurting the animals.

The Mindset - It's Pride And Not Protein

If you live anywhere in north India. You probably will agree with what I am going to say, for people here in rural north India specifically in Haryana, Uttar Pradesh, or Delhi anyone having milk is a matter of pride and not a matter of protein. Anyone who hasn't had milk in childhood is belittled.

A common taunt to weak kids here in North India is "doodh nahi Peeta kya?" ("don't you drink milk?")

And honestly, I have no clue about the timeline of when did this start. Our obsession with a healthy or protein-full diet became a matter of pride.

This is mostly in rural areas, or probably in urban areas too, but with people having a conventional mindset. so, all those who say milk is powerful and gives you protein and strength, I am sure, don't even know what proteins it has.

So if you will ask a 60-yr-old person,

"Why do you stress too much about having milk?"

They say "because we had it".

"So what? You have diabetes and heart troubles."

"This is because of our age."

"But you had diabetes when you were 40-yr-old."

Silence!!!

Therefore, if you have a grandparent at home, who is either diabetic or has hypothyroidism, all the best to convince them to stop milk, for good. A few of them take a lot of time to understand this. And a few of them just don't acknowledge it, at all.

Once, when I asked someone to do it. They just ignored me and behaved in a way that I haven't said that. They thought I am a doctor, I am educated, how can I say milk is bad, and they themselves, must have heard it wrong. Then, when I repeated it, they said, "oh! Nahi Peena ?" (oh! You asked us to stop drinking milk?). "we thought you asked us to HAVE MILK". And laughed it off. It was funny because we only believe what we want to believe, much easier, as compared to something which is new to our beliefs.

Stop Blaming Your Genes

Milk and other dairy products are the top sources of Saturated Fats in the American diet, contributing to heart disease, type 2 diabetes and Alzheimer's disease. Studies have also linked dairy to an increased risk of breast, ovarian and prostate cancer.

(Reference- www.pcrm.org)

Even if you are moderately active on social media, almost all of you must have seen some video or picture of how our Earth is stumbling for survival. And if you are not on social media and you are a little observant of things happening around you, you must be aware of climate change.

A small change in your daily routine can help the Earth to survive, and also can save you and your generations from some of the most common and dangerous diseases. You can stop blaming your genes for all the diseases you get in your life. That is very convenient, right?

For example- let us assume my family has a hypothyroid genetic tendency, but it is only the tendency, it doesn't mean that I will surely suffer from hypothyroidism in my life.

Tendency only means if I do anything that is not medically right, or I mess up my lifestyle, whenever in my life, hypothyroidism (probably) will be the first disease to hit me. There are people who suffer from hypothyroid at the age of 10 years, and some of them can also get it at the age of 70 years.

So, there must be some factors that decide, whether I will get this disease at the age of 10 or at the age of 70. The probability is high that I will suffer from thyroid. But approximately I can save myself from 30-40 years of medical treatment or consultations. This difference, according to me has great value, as it will save my money, time and energy. Imagine if you knew how to prevent these diseases. Big names, like diabetes, thyroid, PCOD, Alzheimer's, heart troubles etc.

IS THIS NOT A LIFE HACK? LITERALLY.

It is amazing how marketing people use tactics to convince us into doing things that may or may not help us, but can surely harm us.

Please tell me if I am wrong, haven't you read about something like this-

"Intermittent Fasting- the secret method celebrities are using to lose weight." It is not a secret method my friends, it is a stupid method that may help you lose a little weight temporarily, only to give you extra kilos afterwards by messing with your metabolism. I don't think you want that.

We, today live in a strangely obsessive world. It is certainly strange when most of us think that all the bodily pains or bone pains are related to calcium deficiency only, or all the weakness or lethargic feeling is a lack of protein or (to give another example) all the gastric troubles are liver-related complains only. But all of this is not true.

And it is most certainly obsessive too because most

of us come to a conclusion and self-diagnose ourselves by just reading something on the internet without getting our investigations done. Or at least give your physician a chance to diagnose it, what's the rush?

An ad on youtube is more convincing than a certified doctor's opinion, please tell me if this is not strange then what is?

ON A LIGHT NOTE, EVER HEARD THE SAYING,?

"What doesn't kill you makes you stronger."

Looks like we have an exception here, because this doesn't go with the milk products, as it might be killing you slowly, and even if it is not killing you, it is neither making you stronger.

THE KIND VEGETARIANS-

Please take no offense to what I am going to write here in this chapter.

Because I guess there's no subtle way of putting these things into words.

Here in India, I have seen vegetarians are proud, that they don't eat non-vegetarian food, because they think that they are kind to animals and do not contribute to the killing of nature or killing in general. And still keep on having milk, cheese, curd or buttermilk and dairy products every single day.

Uncountable, is the number of times, that most of the non-vegetarians will have to listen to the statement- "how can you kill, just to satisfy your taste buds"

Most of the vegetarians, if not all, frown upon at non-vegetarians.

No offense to the vegetarians, but you all are also doing the same, maybe not directly, but indirectly. And then, that is not kindness, that is partial blindness. If you were really not having non-vegetarian food for the sake of kindness only, stop dairy too. If you are doing it for the taste preference, then it is your wish, not judging.

I remember asking someone to stop milk for diabetes, and he told me that he only drinks milk from the cows and buffaloes he personally owns, and not from some commercial dairy company. So I asked him that, then he might not be having milk throughout as the cow will only lactate when it is pregnant and will wean off in approximately a year or max two years.

Then I asked two questions together, what happens after the cow weans off?

And what happens to the cow after its reproductive age is over?

The answer to the first question was not provided because he also knew, that I knew that he was either giving medicines or injections for extra milk production, because he used to sell milk also. And answer to the second question was, "khule mein chhod dete hain", ("we leave the cows to roam around freely in the open"). Or in other words, Disown them when their own purpose is fulfilled. Anyone who owns a cow or buffalo cannot deny the fact that they also administer medicines for the extra and continuous production of milk. And you will most certainly find people suffering from hormone diseases, in these families too, who do not even have any family history of a given disease.

I have met so many people who have zero or no chances of getting high cholesterol or any heart disease, but ultimately, when they still get it and come to us or go to any other doctor, they are confused. Most frequent question- I don't eat non-veg I don't take alcohol and still, my liver is fatty, and cholesterol high, why?

And most of the doctors also are confused about what to answer to this question and dodge the question, or answer in the most convenient way- "must be your genetics".

THE PROUD NON-VEGETARIANS

Again please don't take any offense to what I am going to say next, and also, this doesn't apply to all, there are some of the non-vegetarians who think in this manner.

The non-vegetarian eating population are also proud of themselves thinking that they are too Alpha to be cribbing about some animals dying, "it's natural", they say. Another thing I get from many non-vegetarians that- "lions don't feel bad after eating a deer. Cats don't feel bad after eating a rat. That is their diet, they need that protein, we need that protein."

Amazing how we come up with excuses just to do or have things our way.

So, let me make an attempt to give you some facts about milk or dairy products, in a "believe it or not" kind of way:-

Did you know that milk is actually more harmful than useful?

Did you know that Humans did not start having

milk in search of calcium, in fact, they did it because of a lack of eating options, (details in the chapter- History)

Did you know that at present, it is one of the major causes of global warming or climate change?

Did you know that humans can not completely digest milk?

Did you know that it is making you sick in more ways than you can't even think of? Trust me on this.

Did you know that it has a negligible amount of Vitamin D in it? Much, much less than what is the daily requirement of our body.

Did you know that it also has a very low amount of calcium in it?

Did you know that it is one of the commonest causes of Gastritis and bloating in the abdomen?

Did you know 60-70% population of this world is lactose intolerant, and an additional 2-3% is allergic to milk?

Did you know that it is also one of the commonest causes of obesity and heart diseases?

Did you know it is not the only source of calcium in the world? (obviously all of us know that), having said that.

Did you know, vegetables like spinach, cabbage, and broccoli that are easily available around the world, and almost throughout the year, have much more amount of calcium than milk has in it?

A study done by Dr Jason Fung, a renowned Nephrologist, shows.

Spinach has 450 mg/100 cal.

Broccoli has 387 mg/100 cal.

Cabbage has 196 mg/100 cal.

Whole milk has 190 mg/100 cal.

(more options are found in the later part of the book).

At first, when I read some random article on the internet about dairy could be harmful, I think I probably ignored it. (as far as I remember). But then I was reading a book on how to reverse Diabetes in three weeks by a renowned physician, and a lot of stress was given on stopping all the animal products like meat and dairy both; even then, I thought it could be a little extreme or exaggerated version. Then another book on curing diabetes in one week, by another renowned doctor, that had a chapter on stopping dairy products completely, with, of course, some other factors also claiming to be the actual cause of diabetes. Therefore I read more about it and tried explaining the diet to my patients who were suffering from diabetes or thyroid or PCOS (in a nutshell, all hormone related diseases) and were under treatment for the same, and you know what? It actually helped them.

After knowing adequately about the adverse effects it gives to our body, I think I can safely say that Lactose Intolerance is actually "a blessing in disguise". People who are unable to digest milk have actually a good response to the harmful agents, because not all of us have that ability. Those who do not drink milk lead a much healthier and disease-free life, Irrespective of joint complains or bone-related problems.

I feel for the patients who had come to me to treat lactose intolerance. And now I would want to reach out to them through this book if they ever read this, that I should have asked all of them to stop having dairy rather than prescribing them medicines to help them digest milk properly.

And should have advised them to simply switch to other alternatives. As a human being, I am trying to learn new things every day.

This is not the first book, and I am not the first one who is making an attempt to make the world understand the adverse effects dairy is causing to our bodies and to our planet. But I will try to give you my version of the issue.

Fight Or Flight Response In Mr. Rahul's Case

How making changes in diet and stopping dairy helped Mr Rahul (name changed) get rid of Diabetes he was suffering from since many years. He came to my clinic with sugar levels of around 350-400 even after taking insulin. This was a typical case of diabetes mellitus or Type 2 diabetes. He had a very exhausted look, when I saw him first at my clinic, you know, lax facial muscle fibers, sunken eyes etc seemed as if he had lost all his weight. And when I asked him about it, he confirmed that he had lost more than 20 kg in the past 3-4 years, approximately. He had no clue why he got diabetes, as no one in his family had ever suffered from it.

He owned a small business in South Delhi and wanted to expand it. He took a loan from the bank and some of his friends for this purpose. But the news I believe that shocked many in our country and also shattered his confidence in doing so, the news of demonetisation. He was in huge debt when he came to me, and told me that he got diabetes at that time only. As he explained it to me, he said, when this news came in, it seemed like the end of everything he had worked for, he explained that he felt as if the flow of blood increased in his body, so much so that his heart will explode from it. This was the time he was experiencing Fight or Flight response to a stressful condition. He said he felt a total blackout of thoughts. He was having palpitations and thought he was having a heart attack, which he was not. Palpitations are one of the symptoms of a fight or flight reaction.

Fight or flight reaction was first explained by Walter Bradford Canon, according to which when our body experiences sudden fear or adverse news, it reacts in a particular way, In which our brain is made to decide whether to fight the situation or to escape from it. Hence the name "fight or flight". Medically it causes, general discharge of the Sympathetic nervous system. Basically, it is an adrenaline rush kind of reaction that causes palpitation, and when the body comes under the feeling as if it is under attack, it releases extra energy in the form of Glucose and Fat.

Another factor which is most important to mention here is that he might have dodged getting this disease, had he been adequately nourished. According to me, people who have this habit of skipping meals and have erratic meal timings, due to busy lifestyles or any other reason, are more prone to get the disease when experiencing a fight or flight response. Mr Rahul told me, he mostly had this habit of not having breakfast before going to work.

Both these factors raised Mr. Rahul's blood sugar levels, but he did not know at that time. It took him 2-3 months to realize that it was diabetes, and when he started losing weight, felt weak and lethargic. His first reports, he said, showed blood sugar levels of 500 mmol/L plus. And the physician started the medicines immediately. After continuing the medicines for around a month with not much relief, the doctor put him on insulin, which controlled the sugar levels to normal for a few years. Since then he had off and on been on insulin.

With the help of homeopathic medicines and changing his diet and regimen, with major changes including being able to stop all the dairy products immediately, helped him get off insulin injections within 2 weeks only. The results in this specific case were unbelievable; hence mentioning it here is important. But I still insisted on taking oral medications for a few days and advised him not to stop all the medications suddenly. We gradually were able to stop all the medicines that he was taking for high glucose levels or for Diabetes within approximately 2 months only. At present, he is completely off all the medications for diabetes. With random sugar levels ranging between 110-140, which is completely normal.

Note - We all experience fight or flight response multiple times in our life. In fact, sometimes, several times a day, but this does not mean we all become diabetic. The reason for the difference is your diet. So, in my opinion, if you have had your proper meal or are adequately nourished, there are more chances of fighting a stressful situation than taking a flight. People who have the habit of missing their meals or do frequent fasting, or have erratic meal timings are more prone to getting diseases like diabetes or thyroid dysfunction or any hormonal trouble.

Davidsons, our course book of a subject, Practice of Medicine, in medical college, mentions in chapter 21, that, insulin in our body tends to decrease when we are empty stomach. How and why fasting is bad is a topic for another paper to be written on it. Everyone's body is capable of bearing the stress, be it physical or mental, we all have bad and good days, and all we need to do is, try as much as possible to stay hydrated, satiated and well-rested.

The Strange Case Of Hypocalcemia

There are a few cases that stick to our memory for a long time, because of the peculiarity of the symptoms. Once a female came to the clinic with very basic symptoms like lethargy and weakness. On questioning, got to know that she is a mother with a 3-month-old infant.

Q- For how many days have you been experiencing these symptoms?

A- Approximately a month.

Q- Do you have pain anywhere?

A- No.

Q- Is there any fever or any other symptoms?

A- (smiling) I am a mother, living in a joint family, I have problems bigger than fever or anything like that. I do not have time for that.

Q- Got It! Tell me about your diet, please.

A- I have a very healthy diet, I take care of all the things, I eat carbs and proteins and drink plenty of water too. I have 3-4 big glasses of milk every day. And I still feel weak, I cannot eat anything more than this. Please do not ask me to increase the diet. I really can't.

Q- Haha! No no, I will not. Just one last question and then we will run some tests and see what exactly is going on in your body, to get a better picture, please elaborate when you say, you have carbs and proteins every day?

A- I have a bread toast with a glass of milk for breakfast, then one roti with dal with another glass of milk an hour after lunch, veggies for dinner and a glass of milk before going to bed.

Q- Awesome (sarcastically)! That means you are having one roti, one toast, and a small portion of dal, and a lot of milk in a day, which, according to you, is giving you all the carbs, proteins and mineral vitamins you need as a lactating mother.

Just one more question please, and I will give you discount on consultation. Why so much milk?

A- My mother-in-law says, if you need to produce more milk, you need to drink more milk. That is a universal law. Which I honestly feel is not working in my case, initially, the quantity was really good, but now I feel she (her daughter) is still hungry after the feed.

So, her blood sample was taken, and I prescribed her multivitamins and asked her for follow-up next evening. To discuss the reports.

But, I received an emergency call from her after a couple of hours, that she is having severe cramps and tingling sensation in her fingers and I asked her to go to an emergency room, immediately.

And then after 3-4 days, she returned to the clinic with a discharge summary, which said, Severe Hypocalcemia, a condition of very low calcium levels.

Now, how was that possible? The only thing she was having was milk, milk and milk. Throughout the day, calcium was the last thing she would have been deficient of. Along with that, her vitamin D3 and vitamin B12 were also low.

Her calcium levels were 5 mg/dL at the time of admission, which is dangerously low, and could be fatal too. I had never seen anyone less than 6 mg/dL before. FYI, the normal value should be between 8-10 mg/dL

Strangely, From 8 pm in the evening, she went from well-oriented to almost not surviving the next morning. She told me that she was not able to believe this, as she has always been a milk drinker, not only during or after the pregnancy but since her childhood.

Strange but true.

Conclusion- Do not expect milk to give you calcium. It does not necessarily have all the calcium amount you may require. so, what is all the fuss about? Whatever we have been listening to, or learning since childhood, that milk is the only source of calcium and without it, we will not be able to grow, was all a BIG LIE?

Q- WHAT TO EXPECT, when you are having a lot of milk daily in your diet?

A- The immediate effect that you might experience could be bloating in the abdomen.

Later Effect- Then you may feel that your appetite is decreased from non-milk drinking days as compared to milk-drinking days.

Long-Term Effects- Do not be surprised if you at some point of time in your life are diagnosed with diseases like Diabetes, Thyroid or PCOD, high cholesterol or high blood pressure or fatty liver etc.

Or maybe Obesity or Cancer. Of course, there are other causes also which cause these problems. (www.livekindly.com)

I always give this not so funny joke of mine to my patients, that I have invented the full form of MILK that is,

MILK-Man is Intolerant to Lactose, ok?

Or Man Intolerant hai Lactose Ke. (man or humans are intolerant to lactose or milk).

But jokes apart, dairy products are marketed as the best and the only source of calcium and protein. Which obviously is not true.

Observation and Implementation. Of the facts that I personally believe, most of us know and have observed at some point in life, but do not give much importance to, I truly believe in one thing, that is, we all are immensely influenced by advertisements. Ads are everywhere, wherever we see or whatever we listen to, wherever we go, they are just unavoidable. Or the marketing world, The Media, social or mainstream has the power to influence our thoughts, for good and for bad too. Whatever we see or listen to repeatedly, we start to believe in it, and may also follow it. If you listen to a song repeatedly, you will start liking it after a few times. Hasn't that happened to you? You don't like a song when you listen to it for the first time, but while driving you get that song on every Radio channel and ultimately start humming its tune after some time. And again, after listening to it multiple times, you also start disliking it or getting bored of it after a while. This is the beauty of repetition. Another example would be, If you want your child to do something, keep doing it in front of your child every day, they will start doing it sooner or later. That's how we can influence the subconscious mind of anyone. we see and learn, we listen and learn, and we follow.

So, this book is an effort to make all of us realize that we might be doing something wrong for years and years, on and on, again and again.

As rightly said by someone, "we are what we eat". Everything that ends up on our plate influences our health, so we always have to choose wisely. **Just because the world is doing it, doesn't mean it is right. And just because you don't see the immediate bad effects of something, doesn't mean it is good.**

Male Breasts And Female Beard

Gynaecomastia and Hirsutism. Most of you must be familiar with these terms, but for those who don't know about them, the name of the chapter suggests that now you know what they mean. Gynaecomastia means abnormal enlargement and softness of the male chest, and Hirsutism means abnormal hair growth in women, in abnormal areas like the chin, chest, nipples etc.

Hirsutism might seem more common than Gynecomastia. But it could only be the fact that hirsutism is a comparatively more visible condition and gynecomastia is not. I mean you can easily hide male breasts and it is difficult to hide thick hair on your chin. Whatever treatment you take, conservative or laser surgery, treating both these conditions is a huge challenge for doctors. Because honestly, conservative treatments are not that promising (in this case) and laser treatments are only temporary(in hirsutism) and relapse is more common than we know.

We can relate both these conditions to Insulin resistance. Same cause, but different effects for different genders. Insulin resistance may have different bad effects in males and females.

Let me take up hirsutism's example to explain how it happens.

It's insulin's job to help glucose or sugar to be absorbed by the cells and help us give energy. This means without the help of insulin, glucose can not enter the cell. And what does glucose do after entering the cells? Form ATPs (Adenosine TriPhosphates), which give us energy. So,

When insulin resistance takes place, women produce increased levels of insulin,
↓
This has a direct effect on the ovaries,
↓
Which increases IGF-1 from the liver,
↓
Increased insulin and IGF-1 increase the testosterone levels,
↓
All this, prevents the growth of ovarian follicles through to ovulation,
↓
Leading to accumulation of small ovarian follicles, of size less than 10 mm,
↓
These do not progress through to ovulation,
↓
Hence causing PCOS.

That's why females having PCOS have hirsutism. And the sad part is that it is irreversible. In many conditions you can reverse after changing your diet and taking medicines. Hirsutism is one of those conditions that you just can't cure. Or at least I haven't seen even a single case getting cured. A few cases getting better, but never reversed completely. So, girls, always think before having dairy, or milk, if you start having a single hair growth on your chin.

Most frequently heard words at the clinic:-

"No, I just have only a cup of milk at night, to help me sleep better at night and poop better in the morning" will cost you much more than just bad sleep and constipation. Trust me on that.

Why Lactose Intolerance Is A "Blessing In Disguise"?

Lactose intolerance is an inability to partially or completely digest a sugar called lactose present in milk. Or deficiency of an enzyme called Lactase also causes the condition. But actually, it is not only lactose in milk that is indigestible to humans but also "Casein". Now casein is a milk protein, which makes up 80 per cent of milk proteins, the rest approximately 20 per cent is whey protein, which according to me is a good protein. What makes me call it a good protein is because of the reason that it is digested easily and quickly and helps us massively in muscle recovery, preventing wear and tear of the muscle when we are overusing it. Almost all bodybuilders depend on whey protein supplements for muscle recovery. Some look for it in the natural diet because it is inevitable for muscle building. The importance of whey protein is well known in the bodybuilding world, but on the contrary, the adverse effects of casein are lesser known around the world.

Various studies have also proved it to be a carcinogenic (cancer-causing) protein because of its slow digestion. Details in the chapter- "Problem with milk proteins".

How to know whether you can digest dairy or not is, you can start by completely stopping it for a month, and if you feel your digestion is improving or your gastritis is reducing, that means it was troubling you. Because the degree of intolerance may vary in different individuals. Someone who is mild intolerant to lactose might not observe the effect immediately because of the mild symptoms. On the contrary, if anyone is strongly intolerant they will surely observe the symptoms immediately, and you will find such persons looking for almond or soy milk options everywhere they go.

www.webmd.com, a renowned online portal, says in an article, that 40% of adults cannot digest milk completely, and lactase, an enzyme needed to digest lactose in milk, starts depleting in childhood only from the age of 2-5 yrs. in the United States, more than one-third of people are lactose intolerant, being most common in;

Asian-American

Afro-American

Mexican-American and

Native Americans.

Another online organization named, AAFP, American Family Physician, says in an article published on May 1 2002, that lactase deficiency is present in up to 15 per cent of northern European descent, up to 80 per cent of blacks and Latinos and up to 100 per cent of American Indians and Asians.

It is established that lactase starts depleting in almost all of us in early childhood and continues to decrease as we age. On the contrary, some studies have also proved that few of us adapt to this condition and may continue to digest lactose to some extent in the teenage and even after that too. That may be the reason, why a few of us do not see the immediate side effect of dairy products. And, just to mention again, it is not only about digesting lactase in milk. There are obviously various other issues in Dairy too. Like an extremely weird observation that I had was people who are regular milk drinkers have lower levels of calcium than non-milk drinking people.?

Why do people have low bone density even after a lifetime of having milk? and that too every day, and some people twice a day and a few even more. The reason behind this is milk has an incredibly low amount of vitamin D in it. Even if it has some amount of calcium in it, we need vitamin D for the absorption of calcium in our body and vitamin K too. Let us say vitamin D is the carrier which helps the assimilation of calcium in our intestines and helps calcium reach our bones or teeth, nails or wherever it is required. With the lack of vitamin D, whatever calcium we have in our diet, it is actually being wasted.

Ideally, the recommended daily value of vitamin D is 800 IU per day diet, if we are having little exposure to the sun every day. And approximately 1000 IU if the exposure to the sun is not there. Naturally, cow's milk has a negligible amount of vitamin D in it. But in some countries, cow's milk is fortified with vitamin D, and it usually has around only 100 IU in a cup of milk (around 225 ml), so according to this math, we need more than 7-8 cups of milk in a day (approximately 2 litres) for the proper absorption of calcium, Everyday, For a lifetime, For 7-8 billion people on earth. I don't think we can possibly force the cattle to produce that much milk, and I also don't think we should do that just to reach the target.

So, these are all that the dairy company says about the amount of vitamin D in it.

Therefore, In April 2022, I thought of getting the milk tested for vitamin D, calcium and fats. I arranged three different samples of milk in different bottles, tagged them as sample one, two and three, and sent them for testing from the best laboratory I could afford. Obviously I do not think I can disclose any more information on this topic, and definitely I cannot disclose which bottle had which milk in it. But I surely will share the results with you, which were so amazing and amusing, because that just proved something which I thought was correct, and cleared all the clouds of my doubts that milk has a lot of calcium in it and vitamin D in it.

All three samples had ZERO vitamin D in them. It said BLQ, in the column of the result. BLQ stands for - below the level of quantification. Which literally means there was not even a negligible amount of vitamin D in it. The reports are attached. So even if someone says the milk is fortified with vitamin D, I will never trust it now. All three samples had very little calcium in them, and the amount of saturated and unsaturated fats they had is shown in the results, so see it for yourself and believe it for yourself.

I have seen innumerable patients at my clinic suffering from osteoporosis or osteopenia, who were in the habit of drinking milk throughout their life, and in some cases up to 2-3 times a day. My initial thought process was, there are people who do not drink milk, and if they suffer from conditions like these, that was totally understandable, it made no sense to me for the people who did take it for years and still suffer from exactly the same disease. It was basic logic if people were drinking milk and still getting osteoporosis or osteopenia, or calcium deficiency, that clearly means either milk doesn't have enough calcium in it or they are not being able to absorb calcium efficiently from the dietary sources.

In 2014, One of my family members (who was a milk lover) suffered a femur fracture just by slipping in the bathroom. Sounds common? No, it is not. Why? Because the femur(thigh bone) is one of the strongest, longest and weight-bearing bones in our body. Along with the temporal bone of the skull, which is also one of the two strongest bones of our body, and it does not break easily.

The Human Femur bone has the capacity to bear 30 times our body weight and also has the capability to withstand roughly 6000 lbs of compressive force. So as a doctor, it raised a million questions in my mind like how is it possible to break such a strong bone just by slipping in the bathroom? It was not that someone fell from the third floor, just slipping should not break the strongest bone of your body.

(reference-chapter- Ultimate strength of human femur-body physics, openoregon.pressbooks.pub)

Also, it makes no sense to keep on taking calcium without having adequate vitamin D in your body, as it is responsible for the absorption of calcium, so stress on both if you have low calcium in your test reports. Always get both of them tested together. And please, oh please, go see an orthopedic doctor if you have pains in your joints, stop self-diagnosing and self-treating yourself.

Problem With Milk Proteins

Milk majorly contains two types of proteins, out of which around 80% is Casein and 20% is Whey protein. I would like to talk about Casein here for two reasons largely, why? Because A- it makes the larger part of the milk protein. And B- it is a protein I believe is either lesser known about or more misunderstood.

Casein is a slow digesting protein, in fact, it is mostly the cause of the slow digestion of milk. I will explain precisely how our digestion works later in the book, but what we need to learn here is that anything that digests slowly, creates stress on our digestive enzymes and ultimately stress on our digestive organs like the liver, gall bladder and pancreas. This digestion mostly takes place in our stomach and small intestines, and until any food item that enters the stomach is broken down completely, will not move forward into the small intestines. This is the reason why foods like kidney beans, peas, okra etc cause gastritis and other lighter vegetables do not.

Another interesting fact about Casein is, it is also responsible for the addictive effect milk can have. If anyone is regular with drinking milk or having cheese, know this better, or if you haven't noticed it yet, "try stopping it", you will most certainly feel that urge to have it again and again. Not because of the reason that it is healthy but because you crave for it, The Taste. right? (be honest).

This addictive effect is caused by a component in casein, known as Casomorphins. This component has an opioid-like effect on our brain, which makes it difficult for us to stop it. And when someone says they are addicted to cheese or they cannot sleep without having a glass of milk at night, you should probably trust them. Because It is not a habit or a benefit, it is an addiction.

[Source- www.marigoldfoods.com]

Milk hasn't become harmful yesterday or a year back or two years back. Milk was always harmful to humans, it is probably because of this addictive effect that humans gradually got addicted to and spread false information (unintentionally) about the exclusive benefits without actually understanding it. Or there's another theory that all this genetic engineering thing messed it up only to produce more and more milk. But whatever it is, it certainly is harmful at present.

Just like someone started the rumor about drinking red wine every day, it is good for the heart. I understand it has a few antioxidants that might be a little helpful, but it will come with various other side effects that alcohol gives. This doesn't mean we should be drinking wine every day. Therefore, It is NOT good for the heart, it is good for providing a reason for someone who doesn't want to quit drinking alcohol, and looking for an excuse to continue doing that. And tried to convince other people to fall into that trap too. And believe me, any non-alcoholic will rubbish this rumor, and every alcoholic will love this news, call it a fact and will spread the word as much as possible. Not because red wine is good for your heart, but because he or she wants to cover up for their own guilt, probably.

Sorry to break this to you. But it is for your own health benefit. The most recent report given by WHO in January 2023 stated that no level of alcohol consumption is safe for us. It is a psychoactive, toxic, addiction-producing substance and Group 1 carcinogen. This rubbished all the rumors about drinking a glass of wine every day improves your heart condition, Bro...!! It does not.

I am not a psychologist, I am sure there must be a term for this behavior, too, the closest term in my knowledge is Pseudologia Fantastica, which means fabrication of facts, which is a form of lie and believing in them too. According to Psychology, Lying is a part of normal psychological behavior, can be triggered by feelings of shame and guilt, and is often used to avoid conflict. So, now everything makes sense, right? Anyone who is not willing to quit alcohol himself might use some news articles to prove to others that he is not guilty of that and whatever he is doing is not that wrong. (and any expert in psychology reading this, please feel free to correct this info, and drop me a mail, please).

And, of course, this doesn't end here. Casein protein was traditionally, and even these days also, used to make a strong type of glue for woodwork, because of its thick and coarse properties, and its strength and long-lasting hold. And most importantly, its water-resistant ability is a glue. It's sticky in nature and, in my opinion, extremely adverse.

Also, if you have ever noticed why, doctors advise us to stop having milk when we have a cough, cold, congestion, wheezing-like problems, it is because of this protein, that causes us to produce more mucus. But, all the research claims otherwise, and I have no clue why. But if you have even basic observation skills, You will understand whatever I am saying is true, because most of the doctors still believe this is true. Many pediatricians also, do advise to stop milk when kids have a cough, and wheeze. You must have observed this on your own, even before reading this. Any kid suffering from a cold or cough will vomit out milk more frequently than any other food item.

Therefore, if we consider digestion and other big names in the disease world, milk might be harmful for adults. And if we consider digestion and chest congestion, it is harmful for kids too. So what are we left with? Only people who are addicted to it, only they will be the people who will still have it.

Oxytocin - A Life-Saving Drug For Humans, Still Got Banned. Why?

You are reading this book because you are alive and were born someday. You were born because your mother gave birth to you, and all of our mothers were able to do that because of the help of Oxytocin. That is the importance of this hormone. One of many hormones that play an important role in delivery and postpartum.

Oxytocin, in humans, is a hormone secreted by the posterior lobe of the pituitary gland present in the human brain. The pituitary is a pea-sized gland at the base of the brain and one of the most important in keeping us all in shape and healthy, also performs various other tasks and regulates functions of many other organs directly or indirectly, as it secretes few most important of hormones like-

Growth Hormone, which regulates growth, metabolism and body composition. Growth hormone also is responsible for many Tumor like growths in our body.

LH and FSH- which acts on ovaries and testes to stimulate sex hormone production.

Prolactin- which stimulates milk production.

TSH- a thyroid-stimulating hormone which controls the thyroid function of our body. (you most probably have a level of TSH raised if you are a thyroid patient). The thyroid is a layman-used term for Hypothyroidism because it is the most common type of thyroid malfunction.

Oxytocin

It is also called Love Hormone or Cuddle Hormone, because it is released from the gland when people snuggle or socially bond. It plays an important role also in sexual reproduction, childbirth, and the period after that. Oxytocin is released into the bloodstream as a hormone in response to stretching of the cervix and uterus during labour and with stimulation of the nipples from breastfeeding.

This helps with reducing time and pain during the childbirth, bonding of mother with the newborn through breastfeeding and increasing the milk production for the newborn as it is the most important food for the newborn baby.

But, in most of these conditions, the drug is not directly administered because of the natural production of oxytocin in our body which is oxytocin's natural benefit, but it is also used for another immensely important purpose.

Delivering a baby is a difficult job, I wouldn't call it complicated, but the right word that should be used here for the doctors and nurses is SKILL. Because taking major decisions at the time of labor, requires a lot of skill and experience. Some deliveries go smoothly and some are very problematic. One wrong decision may end up in a disaster for the mother or the child, or both.

Oxytocin is one of those extremely important medicines which is used to stop bleeding after delivery. Because bleeding could be moderate to profuse, therefore it becomes a life-saving drug for the mother. One of the reasons why the newborn is immediately allowed to be kept on mother's chest and cuddled and loved, is because of this reason. Because that increases the secretion of natural oxytocin, which helps the mother reduce the bleeding naturally, but in many cases, extra oxytocin is also given to completely stop the bleeding if it doesn't stop naturally.

Even the World Health Organisation recommended this as the medicine of choice when there is profuse bleeding after the delivery. So any medicine that saves lives should always be the priority for everyone.

WHY WAS OXYTOCIN BANNED?

Oxytocin's retail and private manufacture was banned even after being a life-saving drug because of its misuse by dairy farmers to increase milk production.

According to the famous newspaper The Hindu, an article published on 18 August, 2018, "Himachal Pradesh high-court judgment stated, daily oxytocin injections make the cattle barren and reduce their life span". In addition, it claimed that drinking milk from oxytocin-treated cattle lead to male impotence, early puberty in women and cancers.

After the ban, a few veterinarian doctors jumped into the debate of the ban, against it claiming that there is not enough evidence of its bad effect on humans. As the quantity of oxytocin injected is well below the safe mark.

But that is only the synthetic oxytocin that is available in the pharmacies.

What they probably missed out on is the fact that synthetic oxytocin is much more expensive than the crude pituitary extract easily available in the gray market. Several investigations, led by both media and law enforcement officials, found indiscriminate use of oxytocin in states like Punjab and Haryana. Sometimes oxytocin is used to compensate for stressful living conditions, which interferes with milk letdown. Also, the local pituitary extracts contain, other hormones like Gonadotropins, which also have bad effects on the cattle.

Long story short, as a doctor, even though I am not in favor of banning oxytocin, its use is Indispensable.

It is not the solution. To regulate its use might be it.

The lives of cattle and humans are both important. And do you know what is not important? Drinking milk.

All this chaos could end just because of your simple awareness. And if you are able to stop dairy after reading this, feel proud of yourself, Very Proud, because then, you are not only saving a cow's life, but also human lives.

Those mother's lives who probably need oxytocin after the delivery just to survive and make it alive to a normal hospital room from the labor room are also obviously important. Maternal Mortality is a serious problem; if we talk about numbers, India stands at 129th out of 184 countries addressing this problem. (ref- www.theprint.in). According to an article published in Hindustan times, approximately 45000 females every year are not able to make it to the normal room from the labor room. Yes, that means these many females die due to causes related to childbirth every year, with Postpartum bleeding being the major cause.

Suppose only humans understood the importance of this. In that case, the cattle would live their own happy and free life, the way they want to live, like many other animals like dogs, cats etc., and the industry would not feel the need to produce more milk to sell more milk, and consequently, there will be no use and misuse of oxytocin, hence, the ban will be removed. (The judgment of the legal case of banned oxytocin is still due in The Supreme Court of India.)

Just because you enjoy drinking that one glass of milk to satisfy your taste buds at night, or have a good sleep, starts a chain of events that causes humans more harm, and not that you are getting benefited from it.

Sorry, for being dramatically crude here. At least now, you would not be sleeping so peacefully after reading this if you were in the habit of drinking a glass of milk before going to bed. Pun intended.

What Is BST (Bovine Somatotropin)? And What Is Recombinant BST?

BST is another one of those things which is really controversial in the dairy world. Because the irony of BST is that all the dairy manufacturers find it safe for the cattle, even after being proven to be harmful to them several times. This hormone was banned by Canada in the year 1999 after seeing its bad effects on animals, causing a disease called Mastitis- a painful bacterial infection, involving the udders or breasts of cows. "We really do not know the effects of this hormone on humans, which is one of the reasons why Europe has already banned rBST. The International Agency for Research in Cancer has concerns that rBST increases cancer in humans," And all non-dairy industry-related people find it harmful.

Honestly, I was skeptical about mentioning anything about BST in this book because you may find research giving you proof of both sides, for and against the BST. But then I thought, I will share my view, and whom to trust entirely will be your own judgment. I visited the USA to celebrate the new year with my family in December of 2022 and I went to get groceries with my cousin. There I got to see a new trend which was not in India. Many milk containers mentioned that the milk is rBST free and also said that there is no difference between rBST and non-rBST treated cows.

SO, WHAT IS BST?

Bovine somatotropin (bST) is a metabolic protein hormone used to increase milk production in dairy cows. It was approved for commercial use in the U.S. by the Food and Drug Administration (FDA) on November 5, 1993.

rBST's effects on human health are inconclusive, but it certainly has adverse effects on cow's health. FDA and other American medical associations have repeatedly stated that these hormones don't have any bad health effects and are safe for both cows and humans. But people who are in the dairy industry and also actually care about animal welfare claim otherwise.

Logical observation is now it has been stated in the articles supporting the use of rBST in cows, that its bad effect on humans is inconclusive.

But, it is widely accepted that the use of rBST increases a specific type of hormone called Insulin-like growth factor type 1, also known as IGF-1. And the claim of an increase in this hormone does any harm to the human body is also doubtful. But when you read about the excess or deficiency of this hormone, then you will come to know about two disorders that are caused by excess or deficiency of this hormone. The names of the diseases are Acromegaly and Laron dwarfism, respectively.

Laron Dwarfism- is the name of the disease caused by the deficiency of this hormone, it's a rare disease characterized by inability to make or respond to IGF-1 producing a distinctive type of growth failure, due to a lack of Growth hormone receptors. FDA grouped these diseases into a disorder called severe primary IGF deficiency. It is most important to note that people with Laron dwarfism have very low or negligible rates of cancer and diabetes.

Acromegaly– on the other hand, is a disease characterized by the excess secretion of GH by the anterior pituitary. And obviously in coordination with the point I was making, that is, people suffering from Acromegaly, have an increased risk of suffering from some cancers like colon cancer or thyroid cancer.

Effect of recombinant BST on the ovaries or ovarian count-

It is important to mention, A research conducted at Oxford Academy by Jin G Gong, Tony Bramley, and Robert Webb in the department of Reproduction, revealed the direct impact of rBST on the ovaries and follicular count of the heifers. Heifers are young cows over one-year-old age that has not produced a calf.

The objective of this study was to investigate the possible effect of rBST on ovarian folliculogenesis and ovulation rate.

12 Hereford x Friesian Heifers received daily injections of either 25mg BST (6 heifers) or vehicle (6 heifers) for a period of 2 estrous cycles until slaughter.

Then, blood samples were collected three times a week for the measurements of peripheral growth hormone(GH), insulin-like growth factor-1 (IGF-1), follicles stimulating hormone (FSH), luteinising hormone

(LH), estradiol and progesterone. At the end of the treatment (day 7 of the third estrous cycle), the heifers were killed, and their ovaries were collected. The ovulation rate was determined by counting the number of fresh Corpora Lutea (CL). All antral follicles greater than or equal to the size 2mm in diameter were dissected to assess the antral follicle population.

All heifers had a single ovulation. The treated heifers had significantly more antral follicles than the animals in the control group.

It is of utter most importance that the treated group had a higher concentration of peripheral growth hormone (GH) and insulin-like growth factor-1 (IGF-1) throughout the treatment. Which could be the cause of cancer-like cell growth in our bodies. But, I do believe that more research is needed on this topic. And anyway, a few companies have addressed the issue and have stopped treating cows with rBST for the public interest.

But I don't know about others, because you might not know how this works.

Imagine a scenario in which any mammal, let alone cows or humans, any living being, being forced to produce anything beyond their capacity will certainly be harmful to them. Will certainly give them adverse effects. Imagine any human female being forced to produce 10 times more milk than her capacity, and forcing her to produce milk not only for her kids but for society, for monetary gains. And forced until she is unable to do it, throughout her reproductive age, that is after puberty up to menopause, which counts to around more than 30 years approximately. I am sure you can't even imagine that, no one can because it has never been done with humans because it is cruel, but why it is not cruel to cows? A question we all should be asking ourselves before drinking milk.

We all should, at least once, google the condition of the cows at the dairy farm, or follow the groups on Instagram or Facebook or anywhere else also, who are actively taking big steps in saving the animals in the dairy or poultry farms.

CONCLUSIVELY- Even if someone is able to prove the bad effects of rBST and oxytocin on either humans or the cattle, or not, or even if there is the smallest of evidence that there is a slightest possibility of these causing any harm to us or the cows, dairy should be stopped. Just for a small amounts of calcium or protein which obviously can be obtained from various other sources we all should not be taking that risk. Until the time it is proven bad or otherwise.

Can Humans Really Digest Milk Completely?

One of my very good friends was diagnosed with PCOD, a few years from now. At that time I was still reading or learning about the good and bad effects of milk. Because of my fresh curiosity, the first question I asked her was how much milk does she have in a day?

The quick response was "2 glasses". One at breakfast and another at bedtime.

The next question was- "How many meals do you have in a day?"

And she was even quicker this time in answering - "one".

I honestly don't understand people who take milk as a meal. I mean, how lazy one can be, that you want to avoid eating too?

Apparently, she was working with a big company and had a very hectic job, with a lot of responsibility and stress, having less time for meals and workouts, she was almost always seen with her laptop. She even used to come to parties with her laptop.

She used to drink a glass of milk with bread toast or sometimes, a different variety of seeds in the morning and just a glass of milk for dinner and no food. Only one light meal a day, as she didn't want to look fat.

This means having only one proper meal in a day, and of course, she used to have fruits once during any part of the day and very strongly said that she is highly aware of a healthy diet and has been having fruits every day, and she used to expect that she will be the healthiest person.

But contrary to her expectations, she always looked tired and worn out, and her often yelling used to be, "I am trying so hard, still, I can't work out, I hardly eat anything and still I am putting on weight, I have bad genes and bad job, I can't do anything about the genes but I need to change my job".

This was funny to me because we were always debating about the diet thing. She stressed so much about having the chia seeds and avocados and whatever fancy things that she would read on the internet and could probably arrange those things even if those were not easily available back then.

No offense to people having seeds in their diet, but you have to understand, chia seeds with a glass of milk as a 'breakfast' will lead you only to an unhealthy body type. You have to add chia seeds to your breakfast, and not make 'IT' your breakfast. Seeds are an addition to your breakfast and not your alternative for breakfast. Think of it as a supplement and not the breakfast Or have it as a pre-breakfast. I think all the dieticians will agree to this. I hope so.

And of course, this type of lifestyle, (influenced by wrong information) led her to suffer from hormonal imbalances, with erratic menses and hence PCOS and infertility.

Now think of the above situation in a way, why a

glass of water or a glass of juice does not work as a meal for us? And why does a glass of milk act as a meal?

The answer is simple, milk takes much longer to digest in our stomach than juice or water.

Have you ever in your lifetime heard anyone saying "I will have a glass of juice as dinner tonight"? Or "I will have a glass of water as my breakfast."

I highly doubt that.

Also talking about nutrition- a glass of juice might be much more nutritious than a glass of milk.

AND, a glass of water is much less harmful.

So the good part about having a glass of milk as your meal is, it gives us that satisfactory feeling of satiety, that feeling of fullness in our tummy.

And the bad part is, the continuous spurting of gastric juices creates unnecessary pressure on our digestive organs like the liver, gall bladder and pancreas, and so many things that people are writing books on it now.

Coming back to the question this chapter is named after- Can we really digest milk?

To answer this question we all need to understand how our digestive system works. And you don't have to be a medical or biology student to understand that.

The human digestive system is the most diverse and complex system in the human body, which transforms the food or raw material into the nutrients and energy that keep us alive. Of course, there are a lot of enzymes that play a major role in digestion, but we don't need to remember all those things to learn how the digestion works.

To put it in simple words, It works like any other basic-level system. Food will only pass on to another level if it is passed or completely digested in the previous level.

Largely, humans have 4 levels in their digestive system-

1. Mouth

2. Stomach,

3. Small intestines,

4. Large intestines.

Once the food passes the first level, only then it will be allowed to enter the next level. And our brain very efficiently does that without us even knowing that all this is happening inside us. Like a perfect manufacturing unit.

Whatever solid food we put in our mouth, we can't directly swallow it, right?

Because our brain signals us that while chewing, the food has now become soft enough to swallow easily, and only then we are able to swallow it.

Then level 2, Stomach- when the food enters the stomach, the digestive juices from our liver, pancreas and gall bladder enter our stomach to further break the food as we don't have teeth in our stomach.

Actually, digestion starts while chewing only, and in the stomach starts the process of assimilation of food. When the stomach does its part then, it passes the food to the small intestine. Maximum digestion takes place in the stomach.

Level 3- Small Intestine is responsible for further digestion and assimilation of food, maximum assimilation takes place in the small intestines.

And then to level 4, Large Intestines.

The whole point here to understand is that either we do not digest milk completely or we don't digest it at all. Even if some of us are able to digest it, it is done with a lot of effort or pressure on our digestive organs, which will be harmful in one way or another. Gastritis or bloating is just the tip of the iceberg and only the immediate symptoms. Continuous drinking of milk leads us to suffer from various hormonal and Cardiac conditions.

What Is Common In Thyroid, PCOS And Diabetes?

Thyroid, PCOD and Diabetes are the three demons of the world that are collectively causing more sickness than anything else in this world. If we gather data around the world about how many people are affected by these three diseases, the numbers will blow your mind. In fact, almost every family could be having at least one member suffering from any one of these three diseases. If we had earlier known the cause of these, then there must not have been any need to visit the physician for medication. But now we know what and how it is caused and can be easily prevented without any vaccination or preventive medicine. It is again the effect of the advertisements that we think that only medicines can prevent or cure these diseases which is not completely true.

Of course, stress (mental or physical) plays a major role in when in your life you would get the disease, and another causative factor is our genetic tendency, which decides which one you will get first. But having said that, it is not obvious that we will get it. Most of us think that if our parents had diabetes or thyroid or hypertension, then we will get it for sure. Yes, it does create an inclination towards those diseases, but it is not obvious. I have seen many cases in which people still suffered from thyroid when no one in their family had it ever, and vice versa is also true that no one in the family got diabetes when both the parents were diabetic. Therefore, a lot more depends on our lifestyle, eating habits, sleep, stress management, workout and active lifestyle.

I once had a patient who joined the gym just to tone her body and blindly followed her gym instructor who asked her to stop carbohydrates completely. And also advised her to keep two days a week for only fruits and no main course meals. You can't do that to your body, it requires continuous nourishment to generate energy in the form of ATPs. Stopping carbohydrates immediately makes your body crave for energy. Carbohydrates are the macronutrients that are the major energy supplier to our body. Therefore, that did not tone her body at all, in fact, she started gaining weight after 4-5 months. And when she got her tests, she had her TSH levels high. And after another 3-4 months, her menses became erratic. And on getting an ultrasound done, she came to know that she also has PCOD. This, in turn, led to a sudden and drastic increase in her weight, making her moderately fat to obese. And her conclusion of the weight gain initially when she came to my clinic was what her mother and aunt told her, which was, *"gym join karke chhod do to aur mote ho jaate hain"* (if you stop working out suddenly then it will make you even fatter). That's what most of us think and believe. And many don't even start the workout, out of this fear. Similar is the problem with the concept of intermittent fasting; you just cannot, not eat for 18 hours straight and expect your body to work with the same energy. That's absurd, in my opinion, our body doesn't work like that. That confuses our body, and our brain is forced to generate energy compensating ATPs from our reservoirs. This in turn causes our pituitary gland to malfunction, which in turn gives us the conditions like thyroid and PCOD. I know many dieticians may find this theory incorrect, but you are free to try everything. People who skip meals are more prone to getting hair fall and diseases like thyroid and PCOS.

So what exactly is common between the causes of these problems? Dairy products, most importantly. Followed by many factors like lack of sleep, obesity, sedentary lifestyle, and stress. The only thing that makes the difference here is the hereditary tendency of the family.

All of us know the other causes that stress and obesity or a sedentary lifestyle cause these problems, And this is the reason that makes Dairy the most important factor because most of us do not know about it and have been consuming dairy, believing that it is a perfect meal or food for us.

Can Stopping Dairy Actually Reverse Major Diseases?

I met this girl at a friend's house who had a very interesting point of view on the concept of working out in the gym. Let me call her Ms Funny Bones, as she had a great sense of humor and was always smiling and joking all the time. She used to be towards a non-lean side in her school times as she told me, but was never fat. And she weighed more than a hundred kgs when we were having this conversation, suffering from PCOS, Hypothyroidism and borderline diabetes since a few years.

As she was much younger than me, I had to ask about her family history and her mother was suffering from diabetes and hypothyroidism too. She basically asked me to treat her obesity and help her lose fat with some magic medicine, because she was most concerned about that, and did not ask me about the treatment of PCOS and thyroid because in her view, as she was told, she will have to live with it, her entire life.

My next question was to know how and when all the weight gain started.

"My parents," she said. "They pressured me to lose a few kilograms before I got married. So, I started working out, and probably the workout didn't suit me. Instead of losing weight I suddenly started gaining weight and within a year I was almost double the size of what I started with. I have no clue what went wrong, and I hate working out now."

"Gym also affected my hormones. My menses also got delayed, became painful, everything went haywire."

"It was when I started losing hair from my head and saw them growing on my chin, I realized something is really going upside down in my body, like literally", and started laughing.

"Then I thought it's time to consult a specialist, and went to a gynecologist." She said she suspected PCOS, and advised her to start losing weight. This confused her further, on how she will lose weight if going to the gym made her even fatter.

Listening to this she obviously panicked, and because she had a strong will, she decided to join the gym again and pledged that she will do whatever it takes to lose weight. And she started following what her gym instructor told her to do. And that was 'intermittent fasting'.

It made her lose a few kilos quickly. But, obviously, when she returned to a normal diet, she gained all the weight back so quickly that she lost all the hope and motivation to do it all over again.

This was when we met at a friend's house, and we discussed all the things in detail, and she got convinced to follow a specific diet and start the treatment. I know many doctors reading this may not agree with what I am going to say next, but you will have to try to get convinced. That is, Not only did her PCOS got cured, her menses became regular she lost weight and became fit. Yes, it took more than a year for her to achieve all this. But more than that, now she knew all the do's and don'ts to follow, for life.

Hormones are known to control almost every function of our body, in more ways than we can even think of. Not only physical functions but even mental behavior, our anger, irritability or happiness or loathing etc. all of these are controlled by hormones.

And any disease related to hormones may be directly influenced by milk or milk products. Any other harmful food substance may contain preservatives or MSG or harmful added sugars. Milk is the most common food source from which we can ingest hormones.

Considering all these things Insulin is the most important hormone which if taken care of, has the capability of either keeping you healthy or making you very sick. Insulin has a major role-playing in deciding when or whether you will get diseases like diabetes or cancer or PCOS.

Not too much research has been done to prove the relationship between dairy products and insulin resistance, and many doctors or even experts get confused about it when asked. The common answer is, researchers still don't know what exactly causes insulin resistance, but they mostly relate it to obesity and a sedentary lifestyle. It is also true, people who are obese or have diabetes in their family have more chances to developing insulin resistance and hence diabetes or PCOS.

People or doctors who understand the importance of insulin or insulin resistance are effectively able to reverse diabetes or PCOS. If you know what causes it, you can remove the cause and treat the disease. As in today's modern slang, you call it IYKYK. But if you know and are really confident about it, then you should let others also know about it.

Insulin And Dairy

The relationship between Dairy consumption and Insulin Resistance was ascertained in 272 middle-aged, non-diabetic women using a cross-sectional design.

Ref- This work was carried out by L.A. Tucker, Andrea Erickson, James D. LeCheminant, and Bruce W. Bailey in 2015 and was published online on 29th Jan on ncbi.nlm.nih.gov. Mentioned in the journal of diabetes mellitus.

Participants kept 7-day, weighed food records to report their diets, including dairy intake.

Insulin resistance was assessed using the Homeostatic model assessment (HOMA).

Bod Pod was used to measure body fat percentage, and

Accelerometer was to measure physical activity.

Results showed- Apparently, high dairy intake is a significant predictor of insulin resistance in middle-aged non-diabetic women.

Data from the United States at that time suggested that about 26 million people were suffering from diabetes, with more than 90% having type 2 diabetes.

Danaei et al. reported that the number of individuals with diabetes mellitus has nearly doubled worldwide in the past 30 years.

But more than any research, I believe in observation. I am giving you research proof just to make you understand that I am not the only one who is saying this, it's a proven thing. But even after this, you all should trust your own observation, try it and see it for yourself.

While going through the research, I found many of them stated obesity as the cause of PCOS. In my observation, obesity is not the cause of PCOS; it is the other way round; you get obese after you get PCOS, just like in thyroid malfunction. Obesity doesn't cause thyroid malfunction. Thyroid malfunction makes you obese. Learning the difference is of great importance because when you visit any doctor for the treatment of PCOS or Hypothyroidism, the first thing the specialist will say is, "try to lose weight," but how? Many of them still don't know how to help you with that, hence, they will prescribe you a pill for the lifetime in case of thyroid and will refer you to an IVF clinic in case of infertility caused by PCOS. Or if you are unmarried, then the doctor will prescribe you a medicine mostly prescribed for the treatment of diabetes, thinking that might help reduce the weight.

Not to forget that stress and genetic tendency also has a major role in causing diabetes, but also remember persistent stress mostly doesn't cause diabetes; it is mostly a fight or flight reaction (during sudden/intense, stressful situation) that causes the pancreas to stop producing insulin that causes diabetes. And I may sound crazy to you saying this, but I will say it anyway, that diabetes is Temporary. What makes it permanent is our inability to change our diet, and the correct knowledge of what to do or what not. And for a fact, many doctors nowdays are genuinely reversing diabetes worldwide.

You can easily identify a person suffering from thyroid malfunction in the room, they are always tired and frustrated. Ask this question to any thyroid patient, because apart from uncontrollable weight gain or weight loss, the thyroid has symptoms like Lethargy. They do not feel the desire to do any work, even if they are sleeping well, they will never feel fresh if they have important daily chores to do. As much rest as you can get, you will never have the energy to do a given task. People spend hours hitting the gym, following diet routines, for years and still not getting results no matter what they do, that may be because of dairy products. So if you are trying to follow all the things and still not getting the results, to lose weight, try stopping dairy for a couple of months and try sleeping for 8 hours a day, because weight loss is not only working out, it is also adequate rest or recovery from all the hard work you do in the gym. On the contrary, people who do a lot of workouts and do not get quality sleep might ultimately suffer from thyroid disorder someday.

And why is PCOS depressing, you can ask a person suffering from it. If you are married and suffering from PCOD, you are not able to conceive, even if you do conceive with PCOD, the chances of a full-term pregnancy drastically reduce and the chances of miscarriages increase, which is depressing. And if you are an unmarried person having PCOD, then having erratic, irregular and painful menstruation is a part of life. PMS gives you a hard time coping with day-to-day life and those mood swings that hardly anyone around you can understand. Girls get used to having those painful menses, and popping a few painkillers every month is like a new normal these days. I am not saying they like to do it, I completely understand why they do it, in fact, I am offering you all a solution. The simplest solution. Try stopping dairy products. And also, never compromise on your sleep. These are the two most important things, in my opinion, you need to do for the best-performing hormones of your body. Come on, girls, you don't have to find a motivation to live with it, you just have to find a way to reverse it, because it is possible and many out there are doing it.

Global Warming Due To Milk?

Most of us escape the conversation or argument by blaming the government policies for not taking the necessary action against the causes of global warming and very conveniently say what, as common people, can we do about it? Actually, it is only the common people who can change the face of the world. It's the consumers who messed it up in the first place, it will be the consumers only who will actually help get our Earth back in shape. Any number of policies cannot really or effectively change a lot. Till the time we, as consumers or humans, realize how the business world operates, demand creates supply. Once the customers realize what is right or wrong for the planet earth, supply will change automatically. For implementing this, we all should be aware of what is taking the earth down and what needs to be done. Plenty of research has proven the legitimacy of global warming or more aptly put, The Climate Change. I personally believe in all such sayings like, "Charity begins at home", or "Change begins with you", or "Be the change you want to see in the world", etc. so the first step towards your personal contribution towards the amelioration of the suffering of our mother Earth should begin with your own home, by you. The world will follow.

Global warming is a serious threat, and even if all of us don't agree with it, it is happening and is happening much faster than we thought it would.

Writing this during the time of the Covid-19 pandemic, makes me wonder if we still do not learn from this pandemic, we probably never will. The strength Nature possesses. It's actually a typical NOW or NEVER situation or the effects of climate change may be irreversible. And according to some experts we have already reached the point of irreversible change. We have to realize how helpless we are against the Mighty Nature.

As A.H. Suryakantha states in his book on Community Medicine (a course book in medical colleges) that-

"From the past 8000 years, Earth's surface temperature has risen by 1 degree Celsius only. As of today, it is 15 degrees. From the last 100 years, the surface temperature has risen by ½ degrees Celsius, and at this rate of global warming, it is estimated that within another 50 years, the temperature would rise by 2.5 degrees, and by the end of this century, another 2.5 degrees. A rise in temperature by just 2 degrees could trigger an irreversible and catastrophic state of global warming".

Apart from industrialisation, urbanization, deforestation, vehicular traffic and the burning of fossil fuels, Dairy Industry is also one of the major causes of global warming. Some researchers claim that its contribution to global warming is even more than that of fossil fuels. Others say it's second to fossil fuels. But astonishingly, almost everyone agrees to it. Whether it's the number one cause or number two or number three, doesn't matter, it is one of the major causes and everyone is agreeing to it.

www.skepticalscience.com says, animal agriculture causes around 13-18% of GHG (greenhouse gasses) globally, this is more in developing countries than in developed countries (like 3% in the USA), and combustion of fossil fuel contribution is approximately 64% globally, this is more in developed countries (like 80% in the USA).

These are the two major contributors of GHGs in the world, also deforestation adds a lot to it.

It is not only emissions of CO_2 into the environment that are harmful, methane gas is also the biggest addition, which is even more harmful than CO_2.

Beef or cattle are a bigger problem than other sources of meat. Producing beef requires significantly more resources (e.g. land, fertilizer, and water) than other sources of meat. As ruminant animals, cattle also produce methane that other sources (e.g. pigs and chickens) don't.

Eschel et al. 2014 estimated that producing beef requires 28 times more land, 6 times more fertilizer and 11 times more water than producing pork or chicken. As a result, the study estimated that producing beef releases 4 times more greenhouse gasses than a calorie-equivalent amount of pork, and 5 times as much as an equivalent amount of poultry.

Cheese is the single largest source of saturated fats in the American diet, with increased demand in India also, cheese is one of the favorite things in kids since the past few years.

According to onegreenplanet.org, an article published by Kate Good, in the year 2016, the USA only, produced 196 billion pounds of milk a year. In the year 2013, the USA produced 11.1 billion pounds of cheese (excluding cottage cheese). 1.86 billion pounds of butter, and 1052 million pounds of regular fat ice cream. And this is all just in one country of the world with a moderately dense population.

In India, According to DAHD, that is, the Department of Animal Husbandry and Dairying, India ranks first among the world's milk producing Nations since the year 1998 and has the largest bovine population in the World. Milk production in India during the period 1950-51 to 2017-18, has increased from 17 million tonnes to 176.4 million tonnes as compared to 165.4 million tonnes during 2016-17 recording a growth of 6.65 %.

FAO reported a 1.46% increase in world milk production from 800.2 million tonnes in 2016 to 811.9 (Estim) million tonnes in 2017.

[Reference - www.dahd.nic.in]

Q- What in the dairy business causes Global warming?

Ans- Mainly Two things- Methane produced by the cattle, and usage of an obscene amount of water in maintaining the livestock.

Cows produce around 250-300 liters of methane per day, and this time I will leave the math up to you, calculate and multiply this by around 1.5 billion cattle population of the world. And if anyone is intrigued by how it does that? It is because of the farts, I am just guessing. You would not believe that there is actual research going on 'how to make the cattle fart less'.

Methane not only causes our earth to heat up but also, it is a highly inflammable gas. Human and Cow's farts contain methane and hydrogen which means they can be briefly set on fire too. Now that's a fun fact not everyone wanted to read.

[Reference - www.bbc.com]

Eating vegetables produces lower greenhouse gas emissions yet. For example, potatoes, rice, and broccoli produce approximately 3-5 times lower emissions than an equivalent mass of poultry and pork (Environmental Working Group 2011).

The reason is simple - <u>It's more efficient to grow a crop and eat it, than to grow a crop, feed it to an animal as it builds up muscle mass, and then eat the animal.</u> If cattle can grow muscle by only eating grass or crops, then obviously humans can also grow muscle mass by eating only veggies, thinking only meat gives you strength or muscles is absurd. Many famous bodybuilders are vegans.

So, people who might be skeptical about the skepticism of these facts, may say going vegan is not the solution as its contribution is 13-18% only which is much less as compared to the burning of fossil fuels and transportation, but my point is that it is much easier to go vegan than to walk down to work every single day to refrain from burning fossil fuels. Also, electric cars are the new thing, all the car companies have identified them as the solution for the GHGs and have started manufacturing electric cars, and I am sure, the transformation in the transportation sector is not too far away. Going Vegan is the only most effective contribution you can give to the climate change problem, as it is up to our governments and policymakers to stop or reduce the manufacturing of vehicles to reduce or limit the GHGs they are producing. So till the time they take any action. It is time for us to stop or at least cut down our dairy or meat intake. If you can't really do at least this, I think you should stop complaining or cribbing about climate change. Because always remember, it is not only going to affect only vegans or only non-vegetarians, it is going to affect ALL OF US.

DAIRY AND WATER USAGE

Billions of people suffer from water scarcity in the world. Clean fresh water is an essential ingredient for healthy human living, and according to www.worldwildlife.org, 1.1 billion people around the world lack access to water and 2.7 billion people experience water scarcity at least one month a year. And by 2025, two-thirds of the world population might be facing water shortages.

Let us not think in a way that whether a few countries have this problem at present and your country, or specifically you, might not be facing this, but this is the problem of all and will come to you someday. Earth is our home, not only the country we live in.

This is the most ignored and most "to be taken seriously" issue. Kate Good's article published some numbers also that I would like to share. There are 9 million (9,000,000) cows in dairy operations in the USA alone, and all of them need a colossal amount of water for various purposes like cleaning parlor floors, walls, milking equipment and of course hydrating cows. Cows in dairy are continuously producing milk and hence need much more hydration than a cow which is not in a dairy farm.

A dairy facility that uses an "Automatic Flushing System" for manure, can use up to 150 gallons of water per cow each day. That is 150 x 3.7 = 555 liters of water per cow per day.

This means 555 x 9 million cows (9,000,000)= 4,995,000,000 liters of water used per day by Dairy Farms in the USA alone. That is 4.995 billion liters per day by the USA alone. And the USA does not even have the largest cattle population in the world, India has that. And this much water is used only by just one facility which is the "Automatic Flushing Facility".

Now let us come to Hydrating a cow. As cows are continuously producing milk, they need to drink a lot of water. (87% of milk is water). Roughly estimated, a lactating cow can drink up to 23 gallons of water per day. Let us be a little generous here and round it off to 20 gallons per day.

So, that makes up to 20 x 3.7= 74 liters of water per cow per day only in the USA.

Therefore 74 x 9,000,000 cows= 666,000,000 i.e 666 million liters of drinking water per day by USA only.

And of course, just like us, drinking water is important for every living being, so we can't say it is more important to us and not to the cows. That is not what I am saying, I am just saying a cow is forcefully impregnated, not once or twice, but several times, for making money, and more money.

Just imagine calculating this with around 200 countries around the world, with millions of more cows.

A report by Mother Jones breaks this down, brilliantly, in the number of gallons of water used to grow feed for cows to produce the favorite dairy products:-

- ❖ 1 cup of yogurt requires 35 gallons of water.
- ❖ 1 scoop of ice cream = 42 gallons water.
- ❖ 2 slices of cheese = 50 gallons of water.
- ❖ 1 cup of Greek yogurt = 90 gallons water.

Some of you might ask a very valid question that even crops or vegetables need a lot of water and maintenance for growing. Well, of course, but, there are many other ways in which the agriculture industry is much better than livestock. The most important being it doesn't add up GHGs to the environment, in fact, it helps reduce them. Another factor is the huge difference in the nutritious value of the two. They are poles apart. And in fact, we all know that non-vegetarian food is NOT the only source of protein in our diet. Even if you want to build muscle or go lean. Plant-based diet has everything.

[Reference - blogs.worldbank.org]

What Is The Alternative Then ?

There are various non dairy milk options available in the market, like almond milk, coconut milk, soy milk, oat milk, cashew milk etc. Now also available in different flavors (not advertising but letting you know the options). Also, these can be easily prepared at home, all the recipes are just a google away.

And if you are too worried about calcium levels then I would like to mention some food items that might have more calcium than milk.

According to medicalnewstoday.com, there are plenty of foods that are rich in calcium and may not contain dairy. The article was written for lactose-intolerant people or vegans. Calcium is essential for general health, and according to the National Institute of Health (NIH), in the United States, most adults aged 19-50 require 1000 milligrams of calcium per day. This amount of calcium is present in about three (8-ounce) glasses of milk, which is about 680-700 milligrams of daily milk consumption. (approximate calculations).

A few easily available foods that are a brilliant source of calcium, are mentioned below:-

Chia seeds- yes, it has a lot of calcium in it, but as mentioned earlier, add chia seeds to your meals, do not make chia seeds your meal.

A single ounce or 2 tablespoons of chia seeds

provide 179 mg of calcium, chia also contains boron, which promotes the health of bones by helping the body to metabolize calcium, phosphorus, and magnesium

Soy Milk- One cup of fortified soy milk contains about the same amount of calcium as the equivalent of cows milk. it is important to choose a product that is fortified with elemental calcium.

Almonds– One cup of whole almonds contains 385 mg of calcium, which is more than one-third of the recommended daily amount.

Dried Figs– About eight figs or 1 cup provides 241 mg of calcium. Figs make a great sweet treat and are rich in fiber and antioxidants. Can be taken as a midday snack or can also be crushed into a creamy jam.

Tofu– Tends to be an excellent source of calcium, the content can vary from 275-861 mg of calcium, depending on the firmness and brand. Also make sure to buy tofu that contains calcium salt, which manufacturers use as a coagulant.

White Beans- One cup contains 161 mg of calcium. They are low in fat and rich in iron. Can be added to a soup or salad or in hummus.

Broccoli- It is also one of the commonest sources of calcium which tastes good and can be added to salads and soups. One cup provides 87 mg of calcium.

Sweet Potatoes– One large sweet potato contains 68 mg of calcium in it. It is also rich in potassium and vitamins A and C.

Mustard Seeds- Raw mustard seeds contain 64 mg of calcium per cup. can be added to various foods while cooking.

Kale- Just two cups of raw chopped kale provide about 180 mg of calcium. It is also loaded with antioxidants, which can prevent or delay cell damage. It is also very low in calories, with every 100 grams containing only 35 calories.

Sesame Seeds- Also known as Til in Hindi, one tablespoon contains 88 mg of calcium. It is also rich in zinc and copper, both beneficial to bone health. Results of a study from 2013 suggest that supplementation with sesame seeds helped to relieve some symptoms of knee osteoarthritis. In fact, oil prepared from sesame seeds is also used as a massage oil in relieving joint pains.

Okra- A single cup contains 82 mg of calcium. Also a significant source of protein, fibre, iron, and zinc.

Oranges and Orange Juice- One large orange contains 74 mg of calcium, while a single glass of calcium-fortified orange juice contains 300 mg of calcium.

Is Animal Cruelty The Only Reason?

The point is not only the sensitivity for the animals or cattle; it is also about the awareness of our own health and the world we live in. The adversity of dairy has already been explained in the earlier chapter. But, we also need to understand that for continuous and commercial milk production, there needs to be continuous reproduction of cows at the dairy. Just like humans, cows cannot lactate without getting pregnant. Lactating period of a cow is usually 8-10 months after giving birth, but once they start lactating, the production of milk can be increased many fold by giving them medicines or injections.

Also, just like humans, not all cows can produce the same amount of milk, and at the same time cows are sent in groups to the lactating area, where their breasts are attached to a suckling machine for a given period of time. Even if, at any given time a particular cow might not have milk in her ducts or have less milk as compared to others in her batch, the suckling machine will keep suckling till that particular batch is lactating and this continued unproductive suckling creates infection,with pus and blood. Therefore if any cow doesn't have enough milk and is still forced to lactate, it might not be adding milk to the stock but pus and blood.

And if it stops giving milk, it is sent to the slaughterhouse. But the torture they face at the dairy farm is even worse than getting slaughtered. The physical and mental abuse is inhumane. So there's nothing to be proud of in being a vegetarian.

The average age of cattle, in general, is 10-15 years, but the average age of cattle at a dairy farm is around 5 years. (source- thehumaneleague.org)

So, is animal cruelty the only reason?

No, Human's inability to digest it is also the reason. The level of bad effects it gives on your body is also the reason. Don't only stop dairy because it is harmful to cattle, stop dairy because it is harmful to you, your kids, your family, your health, your environment, your gut, your hormones etc. and many more things directly or indirectly.

If I had to be a selfish person to be consuming dairy just so that it is helping me get calcium, and don't care about how it's reaching my kitchen, or how inhumane it is or what kind of adversity it is bringing to the mother Earth, or that's the only source I can get it from, even then it is not true. Trust me, no one, literally NO ONE is getting benefits from it, and actually, it's the contrary, it's a lose-lose situation for everyone. We get diseases from it, the cattle get tortured for it, and the world is getting hotter by it, so much just to get a tiny amount of calcium which can easily be obtained from numerous other sources. NOT WORTH IT. NOT WORTH IT.

According to jezebel.com, 60 percent of the human population cannot properly digest milk, the rest have varying degrees of trouble, mild to moderate, after having milk products. As a matter of fact, lactase which is responsible for digesting milk in our body starts depleting after the age of 5 years.

Only 5 percent of Asians and 25 percent of Africans can properly digest milk, and statistically, these 2 continents have most of the humans on earth, says Kara Brown (www.jezebel.com)

It is not that in these 5 or 25 per cent of humans lactase does not deplete, it does but, maybe due to adaptability it starts forming again and may help them digest milk a little better than the rest of the human beings.

Also, Lactose intolerance should not be confused with milk allergy because lactose intolerance is caused by a lack of enzyme lactase in our body and milk allergy is an immune reaction. Lactose intolerance can be mild-moderate to severe as most of us do not know that we are lactose intolerant but milk allergy, on the other hand, can be more dangerous, or may be fatal. But people having allergies to milk generally observe the bad effects and stop having dairy at a very young age.

One of my uncles was always lactose intolerant; he always used to have black tea whenever he visited; I never found any difference between my parents and him physically because my parents used to drink milk every day since childhood. And my parents still got calcium deficiency, and my uncle did not. And he never took any calcium supplements, either. So here's another example: you will probably neither die nor have low calcium if you stop having dairy products.

Pituitary Shit-Uitary Gland

First of all, pardon me for the language, but when you realize how much control this little gland has over us, physically and mentally, you will be blown away. This gland is everything.

The only gland we all should know about because this little fellow in our brain controls almost everything, if not everything. It is responsible for the hormone functions and malfunctions of our body.

WHAT IS THE PITUITARY GLAND? (BY DEFINITION)

The pituitary is an endocrine (hormone-producing) gland that sits just beneath the base of the brain, behind the bridge of the nose. It is very small– only about the size of a pea. The pituitary gland is very important as it takes messages from the brain (via a gland called the hypothalamus) and uses these messages to produce hormones that affect many parts of the body, including stimulating all the other hormone-producing glands to produce their own hormones. For this reason, it is often referred to as the 'MASTER GLAND'.

The pituitary gland has two parts. The anterior (or front) pituitary produces hormones that affect the breasts, adrenals, thyroid, ovaries and testes, as well as several other hormones. The posterior pituitary's main function is to store and release the hormone, oxytocin and vasopressin.

In a nutshell, directly or indirectly, it controls almost all of the parts of the body, and, most importantly, it has a major role in shaping our body. Two of the most common weight gain problems, i.e thyroid and PCOD, are caused by, the malfunctioning of this gland. So, if you are planning to lose weight, master the MASTER GLAND.

This gland is like a teacher to us all, if you don't follow a good lifestyle, you will get punished.

THYROID DISEASE- HYPER OR HYPO THYROIDS

42 million- That's the number of thyroid patients in India at present (while I am writing this book), and this is evolving data. Actually, these numbers represent those who know they have thyroid malfunction or are diagnosed with thyroid malfunction because they got it checked because of having some symptoms or happened to visit the doctor. There must be many more who are suffering from asymptomatic or fluctuating thyroid and might not be coming under this study. Many don't even know that continuous pain in calves is also a symptom of thyroid and not only weight gain or weight loss. Excessive feelings of lethargy and feeling sleepy always also could be a precursor for thyroid malfunction. These are very common symptoms that almost all of us feel one day or the other. But not to ignore the fact that it could be the symptom for many other complaints also. Lack of sleep or adequate rest for consecutive days also can give you this disease.

PCOS- Another menace in the modern world, aka Polycystic ovarian syndrome/disease- 1 in 5 females in India suffers from the disease, which means it is even more common than thyroid. There's a huge population suffering from this around the world. It is one of the most common causes of INFERTILITY. And it is only infertility and weight gain which take women to the doctor, and after investigations, they come to know they have PCOS. Other symptoms are irregular menses, delayed menses, Hirsutism (i.e. hair growth on chin), and Acanthosis Nigricans (i.e. a dark black line on the back of the neck).

DIABETES MELLITUS

422 million- that's the number of people suffering from diabetes worldwide, and that too, this figure is from the data published in 2014. This number has increased from 108 million in 1980. In 2016, 1.6 million deaths were caused directly due to diabetes only.

All these diseases, combined with cardiac disorders, cancer etc that might be caused by dairy products are definitely more than any other cause of death worldwide.

Endnote

This end note may make sense if the entire book was not enough for you to be convinced to stop dairy products.

Final thought-provoking attempt.

Everyone knows smoking is bad; it is proven to be unhealthy in various ways. It is a well-known fact that it can cause heart diseases, lung disorders, cancer etc. it can kill you, every pack of cigarettes says that out loud, it's mentioned on it Large and Clear. Still, people choose to smoke. Why?

The answer is Nicotine. Nicotine in tobacco gets absorbed by the lungs very quickly and enters our blood within 10 seconds of our first drag of a cigarette, causing a person to have a pleasant feeling and distracting them from the unpleasant feelings. This is the basic reason why everyone gets addicted to it. That pleasant feeling. And many types of research have proved that smoking even once can also get you addicted to it.

Similarly, alcohol also, we all know it is harmful, to our liver, heart, kidneys, mind etc. still people consume it. why?

In this case, it's Endorphins. People who drink alcohol get that high and happy feeling, there is a release of naturally occurring, feel-good opioids called Endorphins after drinking alcohol, which excites the parts of the brain associated with reward processing. It doesn't matter if you are a heavy drinker or a light drinker. Endorphins release is a feel-good factor and it makes you want more.

Also, according to www.webmd.com, alcohol contributes to approximately 2.6% of American deaths every year.

But this book is not about smoking and alcohol. It is about milk, let us talk about that. Milk has 2 types of proteins in it, out of which 20% is whey, and 80% is Casein. Casein in milk releases something called Beta-Casomorphins after digestion, which can also have opioids like effects on our brain (which is also explained in the chapter- problem with milk proteins). May be in very low intensity as compared to alcohol, as you never feel high or woozy after having a glass of milk, but many people do feel sleepy after having a glass of milk or buttermilk. That relaxing feel or sleepy feel is probably because of melatonin in milk, and the inability to stop having milk or buttermilk is because of Beta-Casomorphins.

There is a fair possibility that you are addicted to dairy.

Maybe that's why having it every day makes it even harder for you to stop it when advised. And I have literally seen people saying, "we are okay living with a disease that forces us to pop a pill for it every day, for our entire life, but stopping milk is not an option." If this is not an addiction, then what is?

Roughly, three to four years back, a married couple came to me for treatment of the ailments they were suffering from, since many years. The wife came for hypothyroidism, and the husband for alcoholic Hepatomegaly (liver enlargement). I asked the case-taking questions from both of them separately (because the husband insisted upon it). With one waiting in the waiting area having no clue about what diet I am advising and what questions I am asking. Ironically, both of them had the similar answer to two completely different questions, when I asked the husband to stop having alcohol and the wife to stop having milk. Both of them were, "won't you be able to treat us if we don't stop having this?"

Hypothyroid was making her obese rapidly, she wanted to lose weight but was not willing to stop dairy. Similarly, with the husband, he was losing weight because of high levels of SGOT and SGPT in his liver report and had a complete loss of appetite.

Conclusion- Both of them were addicted to something. It made them feel low and sad when they were asked to stop drinking alcohol and milk. And there is no comparison between them. Right?

Alcohol is bad, and milk is good. I hope you still don't believe this. Both of them are bad, and maybe milk is even worse.

Obviously, both of them were treated successfully for the conditions that they had.

But, there will always be people who still choose to drink milk even after reading this book, not because they think it is good for them, or they have felt it is good for them, but because they are addicted to it and are probably looking for an excuse to have it by any means. Exactly, like people who are addicted to alcohol or smoking and always find ways or excuses to consume it.

And if we count the number of deaths caused by diabetes, that will probably be more than any other disease in the world. Even more than deaths caused by the bad effects of alcohol or smoking. So, if stopping dairy products is saving you from dying of a diseased and unnatural death, and also saving cows from going through a living hell, nothing is more worth it. Stop Having Dairy Products.

HAVE A HAPPY, HEALTHY LIFE

Sample Description	: Sample 1 - Milk		Date of End of Analysis	: 4-Apr-22
Sample Drawn By	: Client		Date of Report	: 5-Apr-22
Sample Quantity & Condition	: Approx 250ml of Milk in a client packaging is intact without any leaks or breaks			

RESULTS OF ANALYSIS

Sr.No.	Parameters	Units	Methods	Results of Analysis
1	Vitamin D	mg/100g	AGSS/CHEM/SOP/HPLC-04	BLQ

BLQ - Below Limit of Quantification
LOQ (Limit of Quantification) for Vitamin D = 0.1mg/100g

Sample Description	: Sample 1 - Milk		Date of End of Analysis	: 4-Apr-22
Sample Drawn By	: Client		Date of Report	: 5-Apr-22
Sample Quantity & Condition	: Approx 250ml of Milk in a client packaging is intact without any leaks or breaks			

RESULTS OF ANALYSIS

Sr.No.	Parameters	Units	Methods	Results of Analysis
1	Saturated Fat	g/100g	AGSS/CHEM/SOP/GC-08	0.89
Unsaturated Fat				
1	Monounsaturated Fat	g/100g	AGSS/CHEM/SOP/GC-08	0.29
2	Polyunsaturated Fat	g/100g	AGSS/CHEM/SOP/GC-08	BLQ

BLQ - Below Limit of Quantification
LOQ (Limit of Quantification) for Polyunsaturated Fat = 0.1g/100g

Sample Description	: Sample 3 - Milk		Date of End of Analysis	: 4-Apr-22
Sample Drawn By	: Client		Date of Report	: 5-Apr-22
Sample Quantity & Condition	: Approx 250ml of Milk in a client packaging is intact without any leaks or breaks

RESULTS OF ANALYSIS

Sr.No.	Parameters	Units	Methods	Results of Analysis
1	Vitamin D	mg/100g	AGSS/CHEM/SOP/HPLC-04	BLQ

BLQ - Below Limit of Quantification
LOQ (Limit of Quantification) for Vitamin D = 0.1mg/100g

Sample Description	: Sample 3 - Milk		Date of End of Analysis	: 4-Apr-22
Sample Drawn By	: Client		Date of Report	: 5-Apr-22
Sample Quantity & Condition	: Approx 250ml of Milk in a client packaging is intact without any leaks or breaks

RESULTS OF ANALYSIS

Sr.No.	Parameters	Units	Methods	Results of Analysis
1	Saturated Fat	g/100g	AGSS/CHEM/SOP/GC-08	2.9
Unsaturated Fat				
1	Monounsaturated Fat	g/100g	AGSS/CHEM/SOP/GC-08	1.1
2	Polyunsaturated Fat	g/100g	AGSS/CHEM/SOP/GC-08	BLQ

BLQ - Below Limit of Quantification
LOQ (Limit of Quantification) for Polyunsaturated Fat = 0.1g/100g

Sample Description	: Sample 3 - Milk		Date of End of Analysis	: 4-Apr-22
Sample Drawn By	: Client		Date of Report	: 5-Apr-22
Sample Quantity & Condition	: Approx 250ml of Milk in a client packaging is intact without any leaks or breaks			

RESULTS OF ANALYSIS

Sr.No.	Parameters	Units	Methods	Results of Analysis
1	Calcium	mg/100g	IS:4285	158.80

Sample Description	: Sample 2 - Milk		Date of End of Analysis	: 4-Apr-22
Sample Drawn By	: Client		Date of Report	: 5-Apr-22
Sample Quantity & Condition	: Approx 250ml of Milk in a client packaging is intact without any leaks or breaks			

RESULTS OF ANALYSIS

Sr.No.	Parameters	Units	Methods	Results of Analysis
1	Saturated Fat	g/100g	AGSS/CHEM/SOP/GC-08	0.86
Unsaturated Fat				
1	Monounsaturated Fat	g/100g	AGSS/CHEM/SOP/GC-08	0.26
2	Polyunsaturated Fat	g/100g	AGSS/CHEM/SOP/GC-08	BLQ

BLQ - Below Limit of Quantification
LOQ (Limit of Quantification) for Polyunsaturated Fat = 0.1g/100g

Sample Description	: Sample 2 - Milk		Date of End of Analysis	: 4-Apr-22
Sample Drawn By	: Client		Date of Report	: 5-Apr-22
Sample Quantity & Condition		: Approx 250ml of Milk in a client packaging is intact without any leaks or breaks

RESULTS OF ANALYSIS

Sr.No.	Parameters	Units	Methods	Results of Analysis
1	Calcium	mg/100g	IS:4285	158.80

Sample Description	: Sample 2 - Milk	Date of End of Analysis	: 4-Apr-22
Sample Drawn By	: Client	Date of Report	: 5-Apr-22
Sample Quantity & Condition		: Approx 250ml of Milk in a client packaging is intact without any leaks or breaks

RESULTS OF ANALYSIS

Sr.No.	Parameters	Units	Methods	Results of Analysis
1	Vitamin D	mg/100g	AGSS/CHEM/SOP/HPLC-04	BLQ

BLQ - Below Limit of Quantification
LOQ (Limit of Quantification) for Vitamin D = 0.1mg/100g

Sample Description	: Sample 1 - Milk		Date of End of Analysis	: 4-Apr-22
Sample Drawn By	: Client		Date of Report	: 5-Apr-22
Sample Quantity & Condition	: Approx 250ml of Milk in a client packaging is intact without any leaks or breaks			

RESULTS OF ANALYSIS

Sr.No.	Parameters	Units	Methods	Results of Analysis
1	Calcium	mg/100g	IS:4285	106.09

THE WRITE ORDER

You Write. We Publish.

To publish your own book, contact us.

We publish poetry collections, short story collections, novellas and novels.

contact@thewriteorder.com

Instagram- thewriteorder

www.facebook.com/thewriteorder

www.ingramcontent.com/pod-product-compliance
Lightning Source LLC
LaVergne TN
LVHW020446070526
838199LV00063B/4859